Self-Efficacy And Perceived Susceptibility As Predictors Of Condom Use Among African American Males

DR. KARLA NASH

PUBLISHED BY KARLA NASH, PH.D.

Self-Efficacy and Perceived Susceptibility as Predictors of Condom Use Among African American Males

Photo Editor, Jo Ann Nash
Photographer, Chocolate Nash

Paperback ISBN: 978-1-958356-66-1

Published by Dr. Karla Nash
Printed in the United States

Walden University

College of Psychology and Community Services

This is to certify that the doctoral dissertation by

Dr. Karla Nash

has been found to be complete and satisfactory in all respects,
and that any and all revisions required by
the review committee have been made.

Review Committee
Dr. Brandy Benson, Committee Chairperson, Psychology
Faculty Dr. Lisa Scharff, Committee Member, Psychology
Faculty
Dr. Neal McBride, University Reviewer, Psychology Faculty

Chief Academic Officer and Provost
Sue Subocz, Ph.D.

Walden University 2022

Abstract

Self-Efficacy and Perceived Susceptibility as Predictors of Condom Use Among African American Males

by

Dr. Karla Nash

MA, Walden University, 2011

BS, Walden University, 2003

Dissertation Submitted in Partial Fulfillment of the Requirements for the Degree of

Doctor of Philosophy

Clinical Psychology

Walden University

November 2022

ABSTRACT

Human immunodeficiency virus (HIV/AIDS) is a disease that claims lives on a global scale, and correct condom use reduces the likelihood of infection by 10 to 20 times. African-American males are at increased risk for contracting HIV/AIDS compared to the general population.

The purpose of this quantitative study was to determine the relationship between self-efficacy, susceptibility, and condom use in Californian African-American men using the health belief model as a theoretical guide. One hundred and five African American men between the ages of 18 and 35 years were recruited through local barber shops, sports and recreation centers, churches, and social media websites.

SurveyMonkey was used to administer the Condom Use Self-Efficacy Scale as well as the Perceived Risk Scale, and to ask participants about their condom use. Binary logistic regression analyses were used to predict condom use from the constructs of perceived susceptibility and self-efficacy. The model was a significant predictor of condom use among African American men, improving prediction accuracy over the baseline model by 11.4%.

Perceived risk did not make a significant contribution to the model; however, self-efficacy did make a significant contribution where a unit increase in condom self- efficacy scores was associated with 1.06 times increase in the likelihood of using condoms consistently. Condom usage may be more consistent among individuals who acknowledge a level of comfort and confidence with use for disease prevention. The findings of this study may be used to promote positive social change by highlighting the factors that promote condom use, and HIV/AIDS prevention, in this vulnerable population.

Self-Efficacy and Perceived Susceptibility as Predictors of Condom Use Among African American Males

by

Dr. Karla Nash

Dissertation Submitted in Partial Fulfillment

of the Requirements for the Degree of

Doctor of Philosophy

Clinical Psychology

DEDICATION

This dissertation is dedicated to my family, especially my father, Mr. John Nash Sr., who taught me to never give up and to always think positively, and to my mother, the late Mrs. Rosa Nash, who taught me to work hard, be persistent in everything that I do and to maintain a close relationship with God.

I extend sincere appreciation to Dr. Mary Page for her continued prayers and support.

I would like to acknowledge Lemar Slater, whose continued faithfulness was a constant support on this journey.

Special thanks to Pastor Lonzine Lee for your tireless support of my dissertation and your scholarly feedback throughout this process.

Last, but not least, I would like to thank God for sustaining me and giving me the strength to pursue until the end, without Him, it would not be possible.

ACKNOWLEDGEMENTS

I would like to acknowledge my committee chair, Dr. Brandy Benson and committee member, Dr. Lisa Scharff, for their dedicated support and encouragement. I am grateful for your wisdom and your inspiration on my educational journey.

I would also like to acknowledge Pastor Hazel Dawson and Elder Sharon Hill for your prayers and support through my journey. Special thanks to Dr. L. Johnson and Dr. R. Bastien for your dedicated support of my educational goals.

To my son, Chocolate, thank you for your unwavering love and for showering me with thoughtful expressions of love that kept me encouraged.

Thank you, to my cousin Jo Nash, for your positive attitude and for always lifting my spirits.

TABLE CONTENTS

CHAPTER 1: Introduction to the Study

The intent of this quantitative survey was to examine the extent to which self- efficacy and self-perceived susceptibility to HIV/AIDS predict self-reported likelihood of condom use during sexual activities among African American males living in the San Diego, area in the State of California. African American men are at high risk for contracting HIV/AIDS, particularly when compared to males of other ethnic groups in the U.S. (Kennedy et al., 2007). According to the United States Census Bureau (USCB, 2017a), African American men comprise only 5.5% of the population; however, more new HIV/AIDS infections occurred among adolescent African American males than any other racial or gender groups (Stein et al., 2017).

In order to reduce the risk and disease progression among this group, it is critical to understand factors that contribute to condom use in the African American community. The disproportionate rate of disease progression is a major concern for public health officials and practitioners who serve the health needs of African American communities (Laurencin et al., 2008).

Over the past 35 years, since the HIV/AIDS epidemic first appeared in the U.S., intravenous drug users, gay men, and persons that have undergone repeated blood transfusions have been identified as high-risk groups for the acquisition of HIV/AIDS (Deeks et al.,

2013). African American males are no more likely to be members of these high-risk groups than any other ethnic group. However, discrepantly higher rates of HIV/AIDS among African Americans, particularly African American men, have yet to be explained (Fauci, 2012).

Condom use has long been recognized by medical researchers as one of the most effective methods of preventing the spread of HIV/AIDS. Declining rates of HIV/AIDS over the past two decades have, in part, been attributed to an increase in condom use. However, inconsistent and/or infrequent condom use continues to contribute to the spread of HIV/AIDS, particularly among African American males, who are identified as the least frequent condom users (Kennedy et al., 2007). Lack of condom use among African American men has been associated with insufficient preventative education, poverty, and culturally influenced assumptions that deter consistent use during sexual encounters (Deeks et al., 2013).

Risky sexual practices increase the odds of exposure to HIV/AIDS as the method of transmission is attributed to unprotected sexual encounters with infected individuals. Risky sexual behavior has been attributed, in part, to the prevalence of homophobia among certain subsets of the African American community and presents a barrier to care and treatment of HIV/AIDS. In addressing the health needs of African American men who are at risk for HIV/AIDS, greater awareness and prevention efforts are needed to improve health outcomes and reduce the incidence of sexually transmitted infection (STI; Fauci, 2012).

This study may provide insights regarding factors predicting condom use among African American males, thereby leading to positive social change in the lives of African American men who are at risk for HIV/AIDS.

Background

Johnson et al. (2013) and Loutfy et al. (2013) reported a global increase in HIV/AIDS infection rates among women, but there is a paucity of information regarding HIV/AIDS infection rates among African American men. Social stigma related to HIV/AIDS infection may contribute to the limited study of HIV/AIDS among African American men (Nunn et al., 2012). Sutton and Parks (2013) said African American men, in general have limited access to preventative healthcare as a result of cultural bias and racism, which are implicated in poor sexual health outcomes.

Self-efficacy and self-perceived susceptibility to HIV/AIDS are intricately tied to choices and self-worth, which can promote either healthy or unhealthy behaviors (Blanton et al., 2013). Conversely, Kaufman et al. (2014) indicated that self-efficacy, knowledge, and risk perception are not linked to behavior as a health preventive measure. The authors attributed this contradictory finding to possible data error or diminished effect of the study results. Such inconsistency leaves room for continued research that could support the link between the variables of self-efficacy, perception, and knowledge in predicting risky health behaviors among African American men.

The dependent variable of interest in the proposed study is self-reported likelihood of condom use. For the purpose of this research, self-reported likelihood was defined as consistency of condom use during sexual encounters. Condom use was measured by self-reported likelihood of condom use during all instances of sexual activity using a self-report method on a Likert Scale with the following ranges: always, almost always, sometimes, almost never, and never (Hounton et al., 2005). Self-reported likelihood of condom use was treated as an ordinal scale variable. Previous studies have utilized the Likert Scale as a measure of condom use amongst males (Hounton et al., 2005). Sexual intercourse was defined as "sexual contact between two people involving penetration" (Hounton et al., 2005).

Information was gathered via an anonymous online survey including a demographic questionnaire and measures for self-efficacy and perceived susceptibility that were administered to each participant.

Independent variables in the study are self-efficacy and self-perceived susceptibility to HIV/AIDS. Self-efficacy and self-perceived susceptibility to HIV/AIDS were assessed to examine correlations between those variables and self reported likelihood of condom use. Self-efficacy in condom use refers to individual beliefs in consistently using condoms during each sexual encounter.

Self-perceived susceptibility is defined as individual perceptions of risk to contract HIV/AIDS. An examination of the predictive relationship between self-efficacy, self-perceived susceptibility, and self- reported likelihood of condom use is important because condom use has been repeatedly linked to lower incidence of HIV/AIDS transmission among African American men (Bauni & Jarabi, 2003).

In general terms, self-efficacy is individual perceptions of control over life (Alvy et al., 2011). Self-efficacy improves the probability of healthy outcomes by limiting barriers to self-control mechanisms (Bauni & Jarabi, 2003). Bauni and Jarabi (2003) said individuals who reported more self-efficacy were more likely to use condoms. Alvy et al. (2011) showed a modest association between infection risk and depression.

Depression was identified as influential in terms of health-related choices, such as condom use. Lack of self-efficacy was the mediating factor between depression and higher rates of infection (Alvy et al., 2011). Graham and Bray (2015) suggested that the three variables: self- efficacy or lack thereof, healthy behaviors, and infection rates, are correlated in a way that merits further exploration.

A complication emerges in terms of appraisal of susceptibility, or the degree to which an individual perceives they are at risk. Self-perceived susceptibility to negative outcomes can increase healthy behavior. Maddux and Rogers (1983) said self-perceived susceptibility to a health threat can be sufficient to influence engaging in steps to protect themselves. The widely used health belief model (HBM) (Hochbaum et al., 1952) applies to contemporary health concerns and postulates a positive correlation between perceived risk and health preserving behaviors (Jones et al., 2015).

The greater the self-perceived susceptibility, and the greater the perceived threat, the more likely a person is to take considerable action to avoid negative health outcomes. Weinstein's (1988) Precaution Adoption Process Model suggests that individuals move from the stage of unawareness of a health risk, to acknowledgment of the health risk, and finally acknowledgment of personal risk from the health threat.

The Centers for Disease Control and Prevention (2005) said incidence of HIV/AIDS in men who reported using condoms during every sexual encounter was 70% lower than men with a history of never using condoms. Condom use served to prevent transmission of HIV/AIDS during sexual intercourse in seven of ten encounters (Gulette et al., 2009; Teng & Mak, 2011).

Self-efficacy is susceptible to the influences of counseling and education, thus securing its importance as a variable of study (Gulette et al., 2009; Schwarzer & Luszczynska, 2011; Smith, 2013; Teng & Mak, 2011.)

Research by Schwarzer and Luszczynska (2011) supports the potential for self-efficacy to influence health outcomes Schwarzer and Luszczynska (2011) said African-American males who perceive their susceptibility to HIV/AIDS to be low were at high risk for contracting the disease because they were more likely to engage in risky sexual behaviors. Lack of self-perceived susceptibility may lead to increased engagement in risky sexual behaviors, such as inconsistent or absent condom use, in the absence of risk- reducing counseling and education (Brooks et al., 2009).

The rate at which African Americans, particularly African American males, contract HIV/AIDS is significantly higher than many other ethnic groups in the U.S. (Stein et al., 2017). Research is needed to understand reasons why this pattern exists, and what can be done to reduce risks. HIV/AIDS is a deadly illness, and fatal to those who do not have access to treatment. It is also a disease that carries a social stigma (Quinn, 2002).

Although it is true that African American males suffer from a higher rate of other medical difficulties such as cancer and cardiovascular disorders, disproportionately high incidence rates of HIV/AIDS have yet to be fully understood (Brooks et al., 2009).

Prevalence of HIV/AIDS in this population is particularly problematic because of cultural stigma and the associated impact this stigma has on prevention, testing, and treatment efforts. It is important that the social impact of this stigma is recognized, and researchers work to find ways of overcoming social barriers for the sake of providing effective health education and prevention.

Problem Statement

HIV/AIDS is a disease that claims lives globally. According to Streek and Nixon (2010), misconceptions about HIV/AIDS contraction methods as well as development of prevention programs and health outcomes are a worldwide challenge. The problem in the proposed study is that there is a need to better understand the degree to which self- efficacy and self-perceived susceptibility predict condom use among African American men. 18- to 35-year-old African American men living in the State of California are uniquely at risk to contract HIV/AIDS (Funk et al., 2018).

These men have a greater incidence of delayed treatment and diagnosis for HIV/AIDS compared to their Caucasian counterparts (Henny et al., 2012). Low-income status, unemployment, incarceration, and low education disproportionately impact this population and are factors that are also associated with increased rates of HIV/AIDS infection (Henny et al., 2012; Millett et al., 2012). Participants were recruited from this population in order to investigate how perceptions of self-efficacy and self perceived susceptibility predict condom use.

Lack of data regarding best practices for evidence-based HIV/AIDS prevention in African-American men supports the need for further research (Lyles et al., 2007). The objective was to examine the extent to which self-efficacy and self-perceived susceptibility to HIV/AIDS predict self-reported likelihood of condom use during sexual activities among African American males living in the State of California. African American men frequently go unrecognized as a high-risk group, and many African Americans are unaware of their potentially high-risk status. This lack of awareness has the effect of undermining prevention efforts (Henny et al., 2012) by discouraging health preserving behaviors which prevent contraction of HIV/AIDS (Henny et al., 2012; Shepherd et al., 2014).

Purpose of the Study

My intent was to examine the extent to which self-efficacy and self-perceived susceptibility to HIV/AIDS predict self-reported likelihood of condom use during sexual activities among African American males living in the San Diego area in the State of California. Condom use is an effective method for preventing HIV/AIDS infection.

Improving consistent use of condoms may lead to positive health outcomes, such as reduced incidence of HIV/AIDS among African American males (Shepherd et al., 2014). Self-perceived susceptibility and perceived self-efficacy are the predictor variables. Self- reported likelihood of condom use during sexual activity was the dependent variable.

Research Question and Hypotheses

The following research question and hypotheses were formulated.

RQ1: Do self-efficacy in terms of using condoms and self-perceived susceptibility to HIV/AIDS adequately predict, individually or in linear combination, self-reported likelihood of condom use among African American males between 18 and 35 who live in the greater San Diego, California area?

$H_0 1$: Self-efficacy in terms of using condoms and self-perceived susceptibility to HIV/AIDS do not adequately predict, individually or in linear combination, self-reported likelihood of condom use among African American males between 18 and 35 who live in the greater San Diego, California area.

$H_a 1$: Self-efficacy in terms of using condoms and self-perceived susceptibility to HIV/AIDS adequately predict, individually or in linear combination, self-reported likelihood of condom use among African American males between 18 and 35 who live in the greater San Diego, California, area.

Researchers have indicated that health education with respect to HIV/AIDS prevention is less prevalent among disadvantaged groups, and that African American males are disproportionately concentrated among the socioeconomically disadvantaged; therefore, it is likely that the degree of health education that many African American males have been exposed to has been deficient

(Alvy et al., 2011; Davis & Weller, 1999; Gerrard et al., 1996). Health education has been shown to directly influence perceived susceptibility to HIV/AIDS (Alvy et al., 2011; Davis & Weller, 1999; Gerrard et al., 1999).

Theoretical Framework for the Study

The two theoretical frameworks that were used in the proposed research were the health belief model (HBM; Hochbaum et al., 1952) and social learning theory (SLT; Bandura, 1978). The HBM and SLT support the research and build upon the hypotheses and contain features that overlap and are mutually supportive of one another in fundamental ways (Fisher & Fisher, 2000; French & Holland, 2013; Houlding, 2003; Perepiczka et al., 2011).

The HBM is relevant to the proposed research in terms of emphasis placed on individual beliefs as well as shared norms of communities and groups during cultivation of health-related practices. It is necessary to consider a range of factors that may contribute to beliefs related to preventive healthcare. The HBM was helpful in terms of selecting and developing independent variables for the proposed research.

Development of effective health education relates to the application of SLT principles. The HBM was a framework for understanding how individuals and communities act upon beliefs . SLT can contribute to cultivating the desired health outcome and the Health Belief Model can be used to examine the impact on future actions (Fisher & Fisher, 2000; French & Holland, 2013; Houlding & Davidson, 2003; Perepiczka et al., 2011.)

HBM

The HBM is a decision-making model that involves assessing the process of making choices between health-related behaviors and decisions that influence health (Conner & Norman, 2006). This model was established by Hochbaum, Rosenstock, and Kegels of the U.S. Public Health Service (Conner & Norman, 2006). Lin et al. (2005) said the HBM involves four key areas of health-related behavior: (a) individual susceptibility to a potential illness, (b) perceived severity of said illness, (c) expected benefits of acting on a preventive action plan, and (d) perceived barriers to the action plan.

The HBM can be used to predict how risky behaviors can lead to poor health outcomes, including acquisition of sexually transmitted disease related to exposure to an HIV/AIDS infected partner (Lin et al., 2005; Marriner & Ralie, 2005). African American men in the U.S. are at a relatively increased risk for HIV/AIDS (Lin et al., 2005).

The proposed study examined the extent to which self-efficacy and perceived susceptibility predict the use of condoms in African American men living in the State of California. Self-reported likelihood of condom use and self-efficacy were assessed using the Condom Use Self Efficacy Scale (CUSES; Brafford & Beck, 1991).

Perceived susceptibility was measured by the Perceived Risk Scale (Hounton et al., 2005). Any relationship found between the variables of self-efficacy, perceived susceptibility to HIV/AIDS, and self-reported likelihood of condom use may offer insight that may be used to help minimize the spread of sexually transmitted diseases. The HBM was chosen to guide this study because of the perceived susceptibility variable the model includes. The work of Hochbaum et al. (1952) established the foundational relationship between health beliefs and behaviors (Conner & Norman, 2006). The work of Conner and Norman (2006) extended the HBM to healthy behavioral choices by measuring the variables of self-efficacy.

SLT

SLT utilizes principles derived from learning theories (Grusec, 1992). In particular the work of Bandura (1978) has illuminated the importance of self-efficacy in shaping behavioral choices. According to Bandura (1978), self-efficacy is influenced through four sources: (1) the individual's own mastery based on his/her experiences, (2) the individual's observation of others doing the task, (3) social persuasions, and (4) somatic and emotional states.

I investigated self-efficacy in terms of condoms use and self-perceived susceptibility using the SLT by examining reported health behaviors as well as perceptions of susceptibility to HIV/AIDS.

Nature of the Study

This non-experimental, quantitative, predictive survey involved examining the extent to which self-efficacy and self-perceived susceptibility predict condom use among African American men living in San Diego, CA (Campbell et al., 2016). The variables of interest: self-efficacy, self-perceived susceptibility, and self-reported likelihood of condom use, are influenced by SLT. Campbell et al. (2016) said behavioral change can occur as a result of targeted interventions designed to impact self-efficacy.

Self-efficacy is the perception that a behavioral change can be created and prompts positive health outcomes (Montanaro & Bryan, 2014). Self-perceived susceptibility is the individual's perceived risk of suffering negative health outcomes. A predictive design was selected for the study because my purpose was to examine potential predictive relationships between identified variables. The convenience sample consisted of African American men consisted of U.S. residents living in the San Diego area in the State of California between 18 and 35. The sample was recruited by placing flyers and posters at specific venues using venue-based sampling and targeting predominantly African American churches, barber shops, and historically black colleges and universities alumni groups located in San Diego, California (Cottrell & McKenzie, 2011; Warren-Findlow et al., 2012).

The survey was conducted online and promoted through civic organizations in San Diego, California that serve African American men, as well as personal social media accounts (Facebook, LinkedIn, Twitter, YouTube, and Instagram). Social media was used to access this population.

Definitions

Condom Use: Condom use frequency during instances of sexual activity. Frequency is measured using a self-reported Likert Scale with the following ranges: always, almost always, sometimes, almost never, and never. Previous studies have utilized the Likert Scale as a measure of condom use amongst males (Hounton et al., 2005). Rhodes et al. (2017) described 100% condom use as "using condoms during every instance of insertive or receptive anal sex with men and insertive vaginal or anal sex with women in the 3 months before the baseline and 6-month follow-up assessments" (p. 972).

Health Belief Model (HBM) is a psychological model that allows clinicians and researchers to identify health beliefs, behaviors and decisions that influence health (Conner & Norman, 2006).

Self-Perceived susceptibility: Individual perceived risk of negative outcomes. This was measured using the Perceived Risk Scale (Mustanski et al., 2014). *Self-efficacy:* Individual perceptions of ability to control surroundings to create behavioral changes and prompt positive health outcomes (Wideman et al., 2014) *Social Learning Theory (SLT)* is a method of identifying motivational drivers that focuses on operant and classical conditioning learning theories and psychoanalysis (Bandura, 1978).

Assumptions

I assumed that the sample that was recruited via the convenience sampling technique was sufficient to provide statistically valid results for this population of participants because the minimum sample size required for the study was met. I assumed participants understood interview questions, were truthful, and answered questions to the best of their ability. I also assumed participants had access to the Internet and were able to respond to the online survey questionnaire.

Scope And Delimitations

The research involved possible predictive effects of self-efficacy and perceived susceptibility to HIV/AIDS infection on condom use among African American men living in San Diego, CA. Other variables that may influence sexual behavior such as drug or alcohol abuse, or early exposure to sexual behaviors were not examined. The study was delimited to African American men living in San Diego, CA between 18 and 35. Men of other racial backgrounds were excluded from participation in this study in order to focus on the target demographic.

Limitations

Self-reported survey data which involves relying solely on memory, perceptions, and truthfulness of respondents, is a potential limitation of this study (Creswell, 2013). I did not focus on identifying causation between variables. Therefore, this study is limited to identifying predictive relationships between variables. Direct causation cannot be attributed to variables. In no way can findings be used to conclude that independent variables directly influence the dependent variable in a causal manner. The study is limited to determining whether self-efficacy and perceived susceptibility to HIV/AIDS infection predict the condom use among African American males.

Significance of the Study

According to Campbell et al. (2016), African American men who have sex with other men are the group most significantly impacted by HIV/AIDS. However, the current study included African American men of any sexual orientation. Although the incidence of HIV/AIDS has remained constant with a rate of nearly 50,000 new cases annually, African American gay men have disproportionately been affected. In 2010, this group experienced the highest rate of new cases of HIV/AIDS of all MSM. According to Jemmott et al. (2017), the risk of HIV/AIDS infection also continues to rise in heterosexual African American men between 18 and 24 years of age. Quinn (2002) asserted the importance of conducting research on the rate of infection and proliferation of HIV/AIDS in African American males. Quinn (2002) added that the importance of research on HIV/AIDS in African American males can contribute to the development of an intervention to decrease both the infection rate and the death rate.

Significance To Social Change

Globally, over 37.1 million adults over the age of 15 are infected with HIV/AIDS (World Health Organization, 2017). In San Diego, there are approximately 7,123 individuals who are diagnosed with HIV/AIDS, (USCB, 2017b). The scope of this disease suggests a need for systems and structures to support those who are infected with HIV/AIDS. Lack of support structures due to poverty and inadequate medical services continues to negatively impact health outcomes for those who are infected or susceptible to infection (Brown & Lourie, 2000; Brown et al., 2005). HIV/AIDS is a critical public health concern because of epidemiological factors and nature of disease progression (Brown & Lourie, 2000; Brown et al., 2005; Letvin et al., 2002). The degree to which there is a disproportional rate of HIV/AIDS among African American males has been identified. This is significant because of the impact of HIV/AIDS on both lives and health of individuals as well as threats to the general public.

In addition to implications for individual and public health, there are also fundamental questions involving social ethics and social justice involved in this research. The significant disparity between HIV/AIDS contraction rates of African Americans and most other ethnic groups in the U.S. is a consistent finding in research. It is necessary to identify the wider social framework in which this disparity occurs. There are environmental and sociological factors that interact with medical and epidemiological data which contributes to prevalence of HIV/AIDS in African American communities, particularly among men, (Brown & Lourie, 2000; Brown et al., 2005; Letvin et al., 2002).

Globally, prevalence of HIV/AIDS is directly proportional with presence of conditions such as poverty, lack of education, lack of access to healthcare, lack of preventive medicine, racial discrimination, and political oppression (Arguello & Walters, 2018). While HIV/AIDS is a biological disease, it is also aggravated by social factors.

One of the most important factors is lack of preventive education. During the time that scientists have been aware of the presence of HIV/AIDS as a risk to human life and human health, The most effective means of prevention has been health education (Brown & Lourie, 2000; Brown et al., 2005; Letvin et al., 2002). This field of research underscores the relevance of the HBM as a framework that may be used to promote preventive health education (Conner & Norman, 2006).

The most fundamental idea associated with HBM is that individuals were motivated by their beliefs concerning the efficacy of various health practices. However, it is also necessary to determine the means by which correct information can be disseminated in the most effective way. Beliefs that individuals and communities adopt regarding health practices and preventative health behaviors are largely informed by education (Conner & Norman, 2006).

Therefore, provision of health education may serve as a means of preventing spread of HIV/AIDS (Brown & Lourie, 2000; Brown et al., 2005; Letvin et al., 2002). Health education provides the means by which HBM and SLT can be combined. The relationship between self-efficacy and self-perceived susceptibility to HIV/AIDS influences choices that impact health outcomes.

This study will lead to significant social change in terms of self-efficacy and self-perceived susceptibility to HIV/AIDS and predicting self-reported likelihood of condom use among African American males in San Diego, California.

Results of the study involve whether higher self-efficacy and self- perceived susceptibility to HIV/AIDS encouraged participants to use condoms. Thus, results can help guide development of programs involving how to raise awareness and knowledge of condoms and susceptibility to HIV/AIDS among male African Americans in this setting.

Summary

Increased education has the potential to influence behavioral decisions for those susceptible to HIV/AIDS infections. This research involved filling a gap in current research regarding examine predictive relationships between self-efficacy and self perceived susceptibility to HIV/AIDS and self-reported likelihood of condom use in order to address behavioral health decisions and increase understanding of intrinsic attitudes that encourage safe sex practices among African American men. I address the prevalence of HIV/AIDS among African American men. The HBM was the theoretical framework as it relates to self-efficacy and perceived susceptibility.

Chapter 2 includes a literature review regarding the problem of HIV/AIDS infection rates among African American males. I address the HBM and SLT. An analysis of data that suggest a correlation between self-efficacy and perceived susceptibility and healthy behaviors is also presented.

Self-Efficacy and Perceived Susceptibility as Predictors of Condom Use Among African American Males

CHAPTER 2: Literature Review

Literature Search Strategy

Literature review sources included current peer reviewed literature and website data. An analysis of current research was performed to determine the scope and incidence of HIV/AIDS infection among African American males in comparison to global populations. Further research was used to address the HBM, health promotion concepts and prevention models. An extensive review of self-efficacy and perceived susceptibility was conducted to provide a foundation for this research. Google Scholar was employed to locate relevant research articles on the current topic. The following databases were used: PsycINFO and PubMed. Search terms were: *HIV/AIDS*, *self efficacy*, *perceived susceptibility*, *African American male*, *condom use*, *prevention*, *beliefs*, *sexual behaviors*, *risk factors*, *health belief model*, and *social learning theory*.

Theoretical Foundation

The HBM and SLT were the theoretical frameworks for this research. The HBM is a model that is used to identify how individuals make decisions that influence their health (Conner & Norman, 2006). The model involves attitudes and beliefs of individuals as important factors when making those decisions (Conner & Norman, 2006). The work of Hochbaum et al. (1952) contributed to the development of this framework in the U.S. through the promotion of a tuberculosis health screening program (Conner & Norman, 2006). The HBM continues to be useful in research regarding short-term and long-term health behaviors in relation to contraction of HIV/AIDS (Fisher et al., 2008).

Montanaro and Bryan (2014) evaluated condom use preparatory behaviors including condom carrying, discussions of condom use with partners, and condom purchases. Montanaro and Bryan (2014) suggested that the HBM and the Theory of Planned Behavior (TPB) predict and can influence change of health behaviors (Montanaro & Bryan, 2014). The authors compared the effect of an HBM-based intervention and a TPB-based intervention to a control group. Perceived susceptibility and severity to HIV/AIDS infection was measured in a pre and post-testing. The findings demonstrated a significant effect in both intervention groups when compared to the control group suggesting that the HBM or TPB can significantly influence Self-efficacy that may lead to behavioral changes.

Further research to understand potential mediators among the variables of HBM and TPB were recommended in order to better develop an explanatory model for these frameworks and their influence on Self-efficacy as it relates to behavioral attitudes and actions (Montanaro & Bryan, 2014).

Lin et al. (2005) offered an explanation of the four major areas of health-related behavior associated with the HBM. Hochbaum et al. (1952) defined the four areas of health-related behavior: (a) susceptibility to a potential disease or illness, (b) perception of the severity of disease progression, (c) expected gains or benefits of taking preventive action, and (d) perceived barriers to taking preventative actions.

According to Lin et al. (2005), HBM explains and predicts risky behaviors that can lead to poor health outcomes, namely acquiring sexually transmitted infections resulting from unprotected sexual activity with an HIV/AIDS infected partner. Their work is an example of the linkage specifically between perceived susceptibility and preventive health behavior.

Bandura (1978) said a person's actions are influenced by perceptions of their level of self-efficacy. People's beliefs in their own ability to create an expected outcome directly relates to the likelihood of taking actions that will lead to productive outcomes (Bandura, 1978). Central to SLT is the importance of repetitive action and positive feedback in order to improve levels of self-efficacy within the individual.

The SLT is based on a combination of operant and classical condition models. Psychoanalysis was used to identify motivational drivers, to elaborate on drivers of actions taken by individuals (Bandura, 1978). Chomsky (1959) updated B. F. Skinner's classical and operant learning theories and suggested these complex processes, including language acquisition, are not the sole result of stimulus response theory of behavior.

SLT offers a framework that supports established theories on health behaviors as it relates to preventative action to avoid sexually transmitted infection (STI). Ybarra et al. (2013) used SLT as a foundation for the Information, Motivation and Behavior (IMB) model.

The IMB model identifies specific constructs from the SLT model in addition to HBM as a predictor of planned behavior. Ybarra et al. (2013) added that these constructs are employed in the frameworks associated with HIV/AIDS prevention in regard to efficacy by suggesting that learned behaviors and prior outcomes establish an incentive to take action.

Thus, the IMB model provides evidence of increased self-efficacy for preventive health behaviors. Specifically, HIV/AIDS preventive behavior is influenced by knowledge of HIV/AIDS prevention methods, desire to avoid high risk behaviors, and behavioral skills that cause consistent preventative actions.

Crosby et al. (2014) examined the association between perceived risk of STI among a convenience sample of patients from STD clinics across five major U.S. cities. The sample was 59.3% African American and 63.1% female. Condom use was twice as likely to take place when the perception of a sexual partner having an STI was present. These findings persisted across gender and race, and suggested an association between perceived health status, susceptibility to disease, and condom use.

Kaufman et al. (2014) said health behavioral change models are critical to mitigating the worldwide HIV/AIDS epidemic. Kaufman et al. (2014) identified the Social Cognitive Model, Theories of Reasoned Action, and Theory of Planned Behavior as relevant to explaining limiting beliefs and barriers to health behaviors.

The focus of these models reflects the distinction between risk factors faced by specific groups and the impact on variables that form the basis for intention. These variables are those attitudes, subjective norms and perceived behavioral control.

The Multiple Domain Model presented by Kaufman et al. (2014) considers the role of the variables of self-efficacy and relationship status. This model also involves considering the relationship between social environment and self-efficacy by including the variables of race, age, and gender. These structural variables may directly impact health behaviors (Kaufman et al., 2014).

Major Theoretical Considerations

I addressed the relationship between self-efficacy, perceived susceptibility, and condom use in African American males. Self-efficacy as a distinguishing factor between condom usage and condom refusal has been established in the literature (Fisher & Fisher, 2000; French & Holland, 2013; Houlding & Davidson, 2003; Perepiczka et al., 2011.)

Condom use in African American men is positively correlated with perceived susceptibility to HIV/AIDS infection (Alvy et al., 2011; Davis & Weller, 1999; Gerrard et al., 1996). The intent of this study was to examine the extent to which self-efficacy and self-perceived susceptibility to HIV/AIDS predict self-reported likelihood of condom use during sexual activities among African American males living in the San Diego area, State of California.

Kennedy et al. (2007) said incidence of HIV/AIDS and other STI risk behaviors were prominent within populations of African American male adolescents in urban environments. Positive attitudes involving condom use, beliefs regarding health, social or personal connectedness with HIV/AIDS, perceived susceptibility, sexual debut, unprotected sex practices, and refusal skills were found through regression analysis to be predictive of condom use.

Indicators of prospective condom use included condom-carrying, positive feelings toward condom use, health, beliefs regarding condom use, refusal skills, and practices related to unprotected sex. The link between beliefs and behaviors provides a basis for continued research on preventative health behaviors. I addressed links between self-efficacy and perceived susceptibility in relation to condom use. Any correlation between the variables of self-efficacy and perceived susceptibility will offer insight into the impact of these variables on the behavior of condom use among African American males.

Protogerou and Hagger (2016) produced an integrated model of young condom use in Sub-Saharan Africans based on SLT and

HBM. Protogerou and Hagger (2016) addressed previous limitations imposed by other theories, in part due to a focus on single individual level theories. As a result, the research established a reliable basis for incorporating individual behaviors to health outcomes in the field of HIV/AIDS prevention.

The study population of Sub-Saharan African men and women offers a contrast to African American men used in this study. The cultural and socio-economic forces that influence each cultural group likely vary by geographical differences. The model HBM will be applied to the population of African American men in California.

Baden and Dolin (2012) studied the development of a vaccine to offer protection against HIV/AIDS infection. The research acknowledged the results from nonhuman primate subjects were promising but with limitations. The study calls attention to the limited options for care as evidenced by only three vaccines against HIV/AIDS that have been vetted through the clinical trial process.

In the current study, HIV/AID prevention was addressed through the study of the variable of condom use. Szent-Gyorgyi et al. (2012) discussed the fears and misunderstanding surrounding HIV/AIDS during its initial emergence in the 1980s. The researchers pointed out that patients who were identified at the onset of the disease suffered from few treatment options and poor health outcomes. Discrimination in general society and in the workplace stemmed from social stigmas against those infected with HIV/AIDS across various communities.

According to the National Association of Social Workers (2005), the Centers for Disease Control and Prevention reported a reduced risk for HIV/AIDS along with other sexually transmitted infection, by the consistent and correct use of latex condoms among sexually active males. Consistent and correct condom usage is necessary to realize the complete protective effect. A single act of sexual intercourse with an infected partner can potentially lead to STI contraction. As a result, increased value is assigned to prevention methods associated with inconsistent condom usage.

With regard to the incorrect usage of condoms, the outcome of reduced protective effect occurs despite consistent use as a method of prevention. Karim et al. (2012) contrasted populations of sexually active men in New York City with sexually active women in South Africa.

A review of HIV/AIDS prevention practices within each population was conducted by clinical researchers. The clinical research teams provided education on male circumcision with regard to reproductive health in addition to proper condom use. Participants were identified as those seeking HIV/AIDS screening at a local clinic in each community. The goal was to identify best practices within the populations.

One practice was identified as pre-exposure prophylaxis (PrEP) which consisted of an initial assessment of HIV/AIDS risk level, followed by a prescription of HIV/AIDS medications to lower the risk of HIV/AIDS infection. A secondary goal was the promotion of education regarding sexual practices and the importance of correct condom use.

Pappas (2012) reported that condom usage cannot be effective in the prevention of sexually transmitted infection if they are used incorrectly. The research found that condom use errors are widespread, including not wearing condoms prior to the start of intercourse, removal of the condom before the completion of sexual activity, neglecting to allow space in the tip of the condom for semen, and failing to visually inspect each condom for breaks or tears prior to use. The researcher suggested that these categorical errors can result in condom breakage and general condom failure as a prevention method.

Colbert (2012) analyzed two at-risk clients based on their risk for HIV/AIDS infection. An 18-year-old South African woman was contrasted with a 46-year-old man from New York City. Colbert (2012) placed emphasis on identifying differences in patient benefit derived from the PrEP model of prevention.

The PrEP model begins engages with an initial assessment of HIV/AIDS risk, followed by the selection of an HIV/AIDS prevention strategy that is expected to provide the greatest protection. Colbert (2012) reported 51% of respondents favored PrEP for the male New York resident while 49% supported PrEP for the female from South Africa in a poll of 1,115 voters. The study reported responses in favor of PrEP, supporting global education as a natural benefit to all. Furthermore, education drives the promotion of correct condom use as a prevention method and provides people with the ability to make informed decisions with regard to their sexual health and behavior.

Beyer and Havlir (2012) reported reasons for an optimistic outlook for the spread of the HIV/AIDS virus. Beyer and Havlir (2012) suggested society may soon benefit from a series of scientific breakthroughs namely, evidence of an operative HIV/AIDS vaccine and the development of an effective cure for an HIV/AIDS infected patient.

Beyer and Havlir (2012) based much of their findings on the positive outcomes from early implementation of antiretroviral therapy and the 96% reduction of HIV/AIDS transmission risk to subsequent sexual partners. In contrast, the National Association of Social Workers (2005) reported rising HIV/AIDS infection rates among female adolescents, especially among ethnic minority populations. Fifty percent of new HIV/AIDS infections patients are under the age of 26. Newly HIV/AIDs infected patients' number 20,000 annually.

Crosby et al. (2014) conducted research on factors influencing the use of condoms with adolescent men in short-term detention facilities. Crosby et al. (2014) suggested that the most significant factors in predicting whether condoms are used by these individuals are personal, and that direct intervention methods provide the best results to overcome barriers to condom use. In addition, structural changes within short-term detention facilities may also be necessary in order to foster the promotion of safer sex practices among male adolescents.

Sweeney et al. (2013) presented the ethical arguments related to shifting the uses of recorded HIV/AIDS surveillance data. The study examined the ethical performance of health departments that fulfill the role of informing HIV/AIDS infected persons of their status and the health treatments available.

In spite of concerns regarding privacy, the researchers concluded that the benefits of early detection and immediate treatment would contribute to improved health outcomes with regard to HIV/AIDS. Sweeney et al. (2013) reported that ethical regard for privacy can be a barrier to offering options for treatment. The greater good of promoting the sharing of private data regarding health status was concluded to be beneficial and a matter of importance with regard to health care practices and institutional decisions guiding public policy.

Kennedy et al. (2007) endeavored to create and pilot test metrics to measure the effects of a short-term condom promotion program targeted toward young adult African American, urban males. Quantitative as well as qualitative research methods were employed, and two theoretical frameworks were applied. The stages of change model and social cognitive theory guided the study of existing barriers to condom usage. A quantitative assessment of the prevalence of condom-related behaviors demonstrated by the participants as well as the hindrances to program administration was conducted.

Study participants were recruited at community neighborhood centers and surveyed to obtain self-report data on perceived condom-use behaviors. Participants were randomly assigned to an attention matched program or a designated condom use promotion program. The study indicated high occurrence of HIV/AIDS STI risky behaviors in the population. The results of a regression analysis indicated that perceived susceptibility, positive attitudes regarding condom usage, health beliefs, personal or social connectedness to HIV/AIDS STI, sexual (unprotected) activity, and refusal skills were all predictive of condom usage among males in the previous month.

Additionally, positive beliefs regarding condom use, unprotected sexual activity, carrying condoms, health beliefs, and skills for refusal were all predictors of whether condoms would be used in the upcoming month by study participants.

Crosby et al. (2014) examined multiple levels of influence with regard to the decline in condom use among an at-risk population of male adolescents. The population was a cross-sectional sample of adolescent males in short term detention facilities. Self- report assessments were conducted with an audio computer instrument according to standard protocol for self-interview.

Condom use during the last sexual encounter was correlated with other predictive factors associated with condom use or the lack thereof. Additional instruments measured correlates recognized at five levels of causation: personal, societal, peer group affiliation, family and relational. Crosby et al. (2014) found that adolescents below the median score on the Condom Barriers Scale were 3.4 times more likely to refuse condoms during recent sexual activity.

Previous pregnancies, and peer refusal of condom usage were found to be predictive of condom denial. Crosby et al. (2014) concluded that refusal of condom use in this sample was primarily attributed to personal level factors. Direct intervention was also recognized as a significant approach to overcome obstacles to condom use. In addition, structural changes were also noted as important.

Rationale for the Theory

A correlational study design allows the analysis of the relational questions specified in this research study. Self-efficacy and perceived susceptibility have been suggested to correlate positively with consistent condom usage as prevention against HIV/AIDS infection in African American males (Campbell et al., 2016).

The theoretical framework of the health belief model, along with the social learning theory, has contributed importantly to research in the field. Variables of interest, including perceived susceptibility, self-efficacy and risky behaviors are described by social learning theory. Research has indicated that behavioral change can be attributed to direct interventions focused on improving self-efficacy (Fisher & Fisher, 2000). Self-efficacy and perceived susceptibility both impact the individual's acceptance of assumed risk level for negative health outcomes (Kaufman et al., 2014).

Literature Review Related To Key Variables and/or Concepts

Creswell (2013) said survey data is appropriate for implementing a quasi experimental design. The work of Clement et al. (2015) supported the reliability of a quantitative research design with regard to psychological research. Quantitative research methods support survey data as reliable valid modes of inquiry into a subject area (Campbell & Stanley, 2015).

Key Variables

Self-efficacy, condom usage, and perceived susceptibility were identified as variables of interest in the current research. The focus of this research is to expand the knowledge base associating these key variables with each other in a way that may be used to influence HIV/AIDS disease prevention. Self-efficacy may influence the ability to overcome specific barriers to the prevention methods and ultimately improve health outcomes (Bauni & Jarabi, 2003).

Self-efficacy was found to be instrumental for improving depressed mood, overcoming addiction to smoking as well as the ability to implement consistent condom use (Alvy et al., 2011). Self-efficacy is thought to influence self-control, a requirement for the consistent nature of completing a course of action that demands cognition (Graham & Bray, 2015).

Condom usage has been identified as a required, consistent practice for those who are sexually active in order to improve prevention of HIV/AIDS infection. The psychological influences at work in the prevention of sexually transmitted infection (STI) can be understood through study of self-efficacy and perceived susceptibility (Bauni & Jarabi, 2003).

In terms of perceived susceptibility, the knowledge of a health hazard promotes a self-appraisal of susceptibility to a negative health outcome. According to Maddux and Rogers (1983), perceived susceptibility to a known health risk can be adequate to prompt human behavioral change. The HBM (Maiman & Becker, 1974) suggests that the greater the perception of susceptibility, the greater the threat perception which ultimately may lead to a person taking massive action in order to prevent the undesired health outcomes.

Nash (2008) conducted research detailing the gaps in understanding the experiences of African and African American men as they relate to race, gender and socioeconomic status. The works of Johnson et al. (2013) and Loutfy et al. (2013) suggest a global rise in the rate of HIV/AIDS infection among women. Nunn et al., (2012) acknowledged the disparity of knowledge regarding HIV/AIDS infection among African American men in response to the societal stigma affiliated with an HIV/AIDS positive status. African American men have less access to care regarding preventive medicine than counterparts, a statistic associated with predicting sexual health prognosis (Sutton & Parks, 2013).

An in-depth exploration of the relationships among self-efficacy, perceived susceptibility, and condom use may influence the fields of health promotion and disease prevention as well as lead to research that may impact the ability of individuals to access health care (Johnson et al., 2013). Studies focused on HIV/AIDS prevention in the African American community are required to improve prevention efforts of HIV/AIDS and other STIs, health behaviors may be influenced through health promotion programs that can lead to mindset changes in those who are currently infected by HIV/AIDS or who are at risk for the disease (Johnson et al., 2013). Perceived susceptibility and self- efficacy are central to the thought processes that influence personal behaviors that support positive health outcomes (Blanton et al., 2013).

Psychological principles are used to avoid risky sexual behavior and overcome drug addiction (Mason et al., 2013). Effective strategies for HIV/AIDS prevention require improved access to medical care, along with behavior modification specifically in culturally diverse communities (Johnson et al., 2013).

Reporting by Ulrike et al. (2013) suggested that more than 50% of adults currently diagnosed with HIV/AIDS worldwide are female, and new cases of HIV/AIDS are occurring more among females than males across geographic borders. According to Loutfy et al. (2013), other gaps in research exist regarding the lack of care for women with HIV/AIDS, and the implementation of policy changes would be impactful in improving access to HIV/AIDS testing and sexual health care.

The creation of outreach services for women and men are required to overcome inherent barriers to health care across gender lines. The critical needs facing women worldwide are evidenced by the rising rates of infection globally. Any finding that is relevant for improving health outcomes for women facing HIV/AIDS prevention measures, may also impact program designs that addresses the needs of African American males.

Self-efficacy was measured in a study of African American female adolescents as it related to condom use in their sexual partners. Researchers found that self-efficacy regarding condom use was a predictor of condom use (DiClemente et al., 2004). The findings presented a quantitative assessment of an HIV/AIDS intervention and noted the significance of a culturally specific focus in order to achieve desired protective health benefit in the branding of the strategy of content delivery in the HIV/AIDS intervention.

Brooks et al. (2009) studied a Latino male population in Los Angeles, California who self-reported involvement in gang activity and perceived susceptibility to HIV/AIDS. Barriers to condom use were identified as well as risk factors to unprotected sexual intercourse. The authors found perceived susceptibility to be positively associated with condom usage.

In addition, the following lifestyle behaviors were associated with unprotected sexual encounters: sexual intercourse with a person infected with a sexually transmitted infection (STI), exchange of sexual favors for drugs or money, and sexual intercourse with a new acquaintance.

The Latino male population in Los Angeles, California, much like the African American male population, is predisposed to gang membership in instances where poverty, poor family relationships, abuse, poor academic performance, peer pressure are relevant (Brooks et al., 2009). Findings indicated that peer promotion of HIV/AIDS testing was the largest factor in prompting new HIV/AIDS tests. This suggests that perceived susceptibility in this population was linked to changing the social norms and constructs within the gang culture.

Reid et al. (2014) noted that community level stigma regarding HIV/AIDS affected intervention efficacy. In the sample where African American participants comprised 50% or more of the demographic, self-efficacy appeared to be influenced by an imposed social stigma along racial lines. The authors indicated a significant level of stigma regarding negative attitudes amongst Whites and African Americans and perceived self-efficacy with regards to HIV/AIDS prevention through condom use. The study also found that positive social regard of race relations in diverse communities did not influence self-efficacy in racially divided communities.

While the authors pointed out that racial attitudes did influence beliefs and perceived barriers to condom use among diverse populations, further research on racial determinants of health behaviors should be conducted in order to establish whether social stigma affects behavioral change.

Mechanisms that exist across a societal level may provide insight into the interpersonal behavioral choices that are influenced by social structure. Hounton et al. (2005) indicated a link between HBM and barriers to condom use in rural Benin. The cross-sectional study surveyed individuals age 15-55 years of age. The variables of interest included socio-demographic characteristics, perceived severity of AIDS, perceived susceptibility, perceived condom efficacy, perceived barriers to condom use and condom use during the last occasional sexual intercourse.

The authors stated findings based on HBM indicated a high-perceived susceptibility and perceived severity, which did not encourage condom use. The authors noted that a significant portion of participants in the study acknowledged barriers to condom use including a lack of belief in the efficacy of condoms.

Summary

The literature review indicated links between the variables of self-efficacy, perceived susceptibility, and condom use. The sexual health of African American males who were between 18 and 35 was a particular risk in terms of STI and preventative actions that can be taken to improve health outcomes. Consideration of behavioral health models must be acknowledged and steps to improve prevention must be taken.

There are racial disparities with regards to disease susceptibility. Gender differences between males and females within African American communities require additional study, as the gender gap involving condom use has demonstrated. Due to social and economic disparities, the issue of HIV/AIDS prevention is magnified among African American males. Research in this area will offer insights involving risk factors and tools for improving health outcomes through improved prevention practices.

Given the severity of the HIV/AIDS crisis, information regarding improved prevention practices must be readily available to at-risk populations. Ramifications of contracting an STI, in particular HIV/AIDS, can be severely life changing, and unsafe sex practices often lead to the spread of this disease. Increased knowledge regarding its prevention and health behaviors that lead to safe sex practices including Self-efficacy and perceived susceptibility should be widely addressed. This research is limited in terms of scope of impact but is designed to offer insight regarding these aspects of health behaviors.

The gap in literature that I attempted to address was the extent to which self-efficacy and perceived susceptibility predict condom use among African American men living in San Diego, CA. Although HIV/AIDS prevention methods rely heavily on consistent and correct condom usage (Johnson et al., 2013), psychological factors contributing to the practice are critical in terms of predicting condom use. Self-efficacy and perceived susceptibility play integral roles in terms of predicting health related behaviors such as condom use. This literature review involved addressing the impact of these variables on health status (Kaufman et al., 2014).

HIV/AIDS prevention methods are targeted to diverse populations based on identifiable characteristics in order to promote healthy behavioral choices (Reid et al., 2014). Self-efficacy and perceived susceptibility can indicate likelihood of risky sexual behaviors among populations. Further study of links between health behavior and disease prevention offers a novel approach to addressing the HIV/AIDS global epidemic (Streek & Nixon, 2010).

Research in this area may lead to improved health prevention strategies which may ultimately help mitigate HIV/AIDS among African American males. Understanding the impact of self-efficacy and perceived susceptibility may lead to insights regarding cultural belief practices within this population and aid in terms of prevention of HIV/AIDS and other STIs. It is my desire that study outcomes may assist in the design of health promotion programs that offer preventive health skills to African American males.

A detailed discussion of the research approach for this study, study population, and methods for recruiting participants are presented in Chapter 3. The chapter includes data collection procedures, research analysis of findings and correlational measures, an explanation of the survey process, and ethical protection of human subjects.

CHAPTER 3: Methodology

THE AIM of this nonexperimental quantitative predictive study was to examine whether self-efficacy and self-perceived susceptibility to HIV/AIDS predict condom use in African American men in the San Diego area. As infection rates of HIV/AIDS continue to rise among African American men (Campbell et al., 2016), there is a need for improved prevention methods. Self-efficacy and perceived susceptibility were examined as possible predictors of condom use in this population. Condom use is a reliable method of HIV/AIDS prevention, and increased use may reduce infection rates (Campbell et al., 2016).

This chapter includes a rationale for the research design and population of interest. The research sampling approach and recruitment strategy are also presented. Finally, a discussion of significant variables, approaches to data collection and analysis, and ethical considerations and threats to validity are addressed.

The HBM was used to explain how healthcare decisions and behaviors influence health outcomes, and describe how beliefs and attitudes predict healthcare behavior. The HBM was used as the framework for the study to define beliefs and actions that may predict condom use.

According to Lin et al. (2005), the HBM offers an explanation and prediction of risky behaviors that can lead to poor health outcomes. The outcome of interest in their research was acquisition of sexually transmitted disease after participation in unprotected sexual behavior with an HIV/AIDS positive individual (Lin et al., 2005). Although the current study was not focused on the contraction of an STD, the behavioral practice of condom use was closely associated to preventing sexually transmitted disease in the research by Lin et al. (2005).

Research Design and Rationale

A quantitative nonexperimental predictive design was used to assess whether self-efficacy and self-perceived susceptibility to HIV/AIDS predict self-reported likelihood of condom use among 18- to 35-year-old African American males who live in the San Diego area. A quantitative as opposed to qualitative approach was employed in the study because variables were numerically measured using survey instruments. The quantitative approach allows for objective analysis to determine potential predictive relationships between variables. A nonexperimental design was selected for the study because participants were not randomly assigned to control and intervention groups.

Moreover, there were no interventions involved in the study. Participants were asked to respond to the survey instrument based on their current experiences and practices. A predictive design was employed because the focus of the analyses was to determine predictive relationships between independent variables (self-efficacy and self-perceived susceptibility to HIV/AIDS) and the dependent variable (self-reported likelihood of condom use). A survey method was used to gather data prospectively. The HBM and SLT were used as theoretical frameworks for this research.

Fisher and Fisher (2000) said direct interventions that involve improving self-efficacy can result in behavioral change. Self-efficacy and perceived susceptibility both impact acceptance of assumptive risks related to negative health outcomes based on specific preventative actions (Kaufman et al., 2014). I examined whether self-efficacy and/or self-perceived susceptibility predict self-reported likelihood of condom use among African American males who were 18 to 35 in San Diego, CA using a planned ordinal logistic regression analysis.

Rationale

This study involved examining potential predictive relationships between self-efficacy, perceived susceptibility to HIV/AIDS, and self-reported likelihood of condom use among African American men between 18 and 35 who live in the San Diego area. A convenience sample was used which was aimed at recruiting individuals with specific demographic characteristics in terms of gender, ethnicity, and age (Uccelli et al., 2016).

Research was not intended to offer claims of causation; my purpose was to identify behaviors and assess associations between variables within this population. All variables that were used in this research were measured quantitatively using valid and reliable instruments. Therefore, a quantitative survey design was deemed the best way to test hypotheses that were developed for this study. Independent variables were both scored on interval scales, and the dependent variable (condom use) was an ordinal variable.

Therefore, an ordinal logistic regression equation was used to determine if independent variables significantly predicted the dependent variable.

Using surveys for data collection provides a low-cost method that allows for the collection of data from a large sample. The implementation of the online data collection software such as Survey Monkey diminishes the time and resource consumption associated with data collection. The nature of online surveys allows any respondents to access the surveys anonymously at any hour and allows participants from across California to participate in the research. It also ensures that each participant's responses will be anonymous, which encourages earnest and truthful responses to the questionnaires (Uccelli et al., 2016).

Methodology

Population

The population of interest for this study was African American biological men who were between 18 and 35 and resided in the San Diego, CA area and could read and respond to questionnaires in English. African American men of all sexual orientations and education levels were invited to participate.

African American men represent 6.1% of the total U.S. population (USCB, 2017a). In San Diego, there are about 47,380 African American males. The population of African American men in San Diego is disproportionately affected by HIV/AIDS, with higher incidence rates as well as delayed treatment compared to other populations (Henny et al., 2012).

Higher HIV/AIDS infection rates have been associated with poverty wages, lack of employment, low education, and high incarceration rates (Henry et al., 2012; Millett et al., 2012).

Further, dearth of evidence-based HIV/AIDS prevention measures addressing concerns of this population supports the need for ongoing research (Lyles et al., 2007).

Sampling Procedure

The sampling plan was to recruit a convenience sample of 18- to 35-year-old African American biological men using four methods. First, networks of predominantly African American churches as well as historically Black colleges and universities in the San Diego area were contacted with invitations to take part in this study (see Appendix A).

Second, flyers and posters with tear off tabs describing the survey and providing the URL that contained surveys were placed at different venues in San Diego (see Appendix E). Specifically, participants were recruited within a 26-mile radius of the city center of San Diego (see Appendix F). According to Warren-Findlow et al. (2012), Barbershops and churches or faith-based communities are reliable sources of research participants.

Third, notices and posts were placed on Facebook social media platforms promoting local African America themed clubs and organizations throughout the San Diego area (see Appendix G). Lastly, the University Participant Pool was used to allow for additional engagement with this target audience.

Sample size calculations for ordinal logistic regression was complex. The sample size calculation program G*Power v3.1.0 was used to determine the minimum number of samples for the study. In the sample size calculation, I used a power of 80%, medium effect size of .5, two-tailed logistics regression, and a significance level of .05. Results of this sample size calculation were used to determine a minimum sample of 113 participants.

Data Collection Procedures

Data were collected using the SurveyMonkey (SurveyMonkey Inc., San Mateo, CA) platform. Study measures could be accessed via personal mobile devices of participants that are not limited to tablet computers, laptop computers, Internet-connected smartphones, and computers. Each participant was provided with an electronic statement of consent form stating the risks of participating in this research. Individuals were required to acknowledge that they meet the inclusion criteria of being an African American biological man, aged 18 to 35 years old who is sexually active and a resident of San Diego, California prior to being allowed access to the survey questions.

A list of screening questions was provided to participants prior to accessing the survey questions. Once participants began the questionnaire, each question was answered sequentially in order to complete the survey accurately and as designed. The survey data was anonymous, and no IP addresses or identifying information was collected.

The survey participants were provided an email address dedicated to this research in order to contact me for more information regarding the study. The email served as a point of contact should the participant desire to learn the results of the study or if additional resources for behavioral health and HIV/AIDS services are needed, and all emails were deleted when the study is concluded.

Demographic Questionnaire

Demographic data was collected using a researcher-designed demographic questionnaire included in the online survey in order to obtain descriptive characteristics of the population through the use of a demographics form included in Appendix B. Age in years and highest level of education as well as sexual orientation, number of partners currently, and self reported likelihood of sexual activity per week were all collected.

CUSES

The CUSES was based on the National Institute of Mental Health Multi-site condom use self-efficacy scale. The CUSES includes 26 items related to self-efficacy with regard to condom use. This instrument has a Cronbach's alpha value of 0.94 as a measure of internal consistency at the .05 level of significance (Brafford & Beck, 1991).

Moreover, CUSES was determined as valid with a significant correlation with other instruments on condom use scales ($r = .51$ to .55, p-values $<.05$). Although the CUSES has not been widely used to date, it appears to be the best scale available that is also associated with attitudes regarding condom use. The CUSES possesses adequate internal consistency and its summary score is correlated with attitudes toward condoms (Forsyth et al., 1997). The time required to complete the measure was approximately five to ten minutes. The CUSES uses a 5-point Likert scale in which responses range from "strongly agree" to "strongly disagree." The total score for the 26 items was used to represent the self-efficacy variable. Higher scores indicate a higher perception of condom use efficacy. Sample statements include "I feel confident in my ability to use a condom correctly" and "I feel confident in my ability to suggest using condoms with a new partner." The responses of participants will be numerically scored. The measure was considered as interval data.

Perceived Risk Scale

The Perceived Risk Scale measures the perception of HIV/AIDS risk through the response to six statements, scored on a six-point Likert scale (Hounton et al., 2005).

The Perceived Risk Scale reports a Cronbach's alpha of 0.80 as a measure internal consistency at the .05 level of significance (Hounton et al., 2005). In addition, the scale has shown strong concurrent validity which was supported with a high positive association with depression and negative association with life satisfaction (Lifshitz et al., 2016). Respondents completed the questionnaire in three to five minutes.

Condom Use

Condom use was measured by self-reported likelihood of use during all instances of sexual activity using a self-report method using a Likert Scale with the following ranges: always, almost always, sometimes, almost never, and never.

Previous studies have utilized the Likert Scale as a measure of condom use in men (Hounton et al., 2005). The self-reported likelihood of use variable is an ordinal scale with 0 as never, 1 as almost never, 2 as sometimes, 3 as almost always, and 4 as always.

Data Analysis Plan

All data gathered in the study was imported to SPSS v24.0.

Descriptive statistics were used to present the characteristics of study participants. Frequencies and percentages were used to present nominal demographic characteristics. For the study variables, interval scale variables such as the self-efficacy and self-perceived susceptibility to HIV/AIDS were presented using descriptive statistics. A dichotomous logistic regression analysis was used to determine if there is a significant predictive relationship between the independent and dependent variables. However, the original data analysis plan was for an ordinal regression.

The predictor variables were self-perceived susceptibility and self-efficacy while the criterion variable was the self-reported likelihood of condom use among the participants. The self-reported likelihood of condom use was measured using an ordinal scale. An ordinal logistic regression was planned, because the criterion variable was an ordinal scale, and the goal of the study was to investigate potential predictive relationships between variables.

Therefore, an ordinal logistic regression was originally deemed as appropriate. The originally planned analysis, an Ordinal logistic regression analysis was deemed useful in measuring the potential associations between quantitative variables and in predicting scores on one ordinal variable using multiple other variables (Laerd Statistics, 2018).

The assumptions of this statistical test involved (a) one dependent variable, measured on an ordinal scale; (b) at least one independent (continuous, ordinal or categorical) variable; (c) no multicollinearity (the independent variables are not correlated with each other); and (d) proportional odds (the effects of the independent variables are consistent across the different thresholds or splits between categories of the ordinal dependent variable). Ordinal scale data in which information is collected via survey response can be used to develop a model to describe the relationship between factors (McCullagh, 1980). The assumptions were tested using statistical tests such as calculating the VIF for multicollinearity and the Levene's test for equal variances.

SPSS was used to calculate the test for parallel lines to determine if the proportional odds assumptions are met. If any of these assumptions were violated then the forecasts, confidence intervals, and the insights yielded by a regression model may be inefficient, seriously biased or misleading. If the multicollinearity assumption was violated, the variables were transformed using the appropriate transformation and tested again. If the proportional odds assumption were not met, separate regression equations will be calculated for each of the two independent variables (Laerd

Statistics, 2018). The following research questions and hypotheses will be explored in the research study:

RQ1: Do self-efficacy in terms of using condoms and self-perceived susceptibility to HIV/AIDS adequately predict, individually or in linear combination, self-reported likelihood of condom use among African American males between 18 and 35 who live in the greater San Diego, California area?

H01: Self-efficacy in terms of using condoms and self-perceived susceptibility to HIV/AIDS do not adequately predict, individually or in linear combination, self-reported likelihood of condom use among African American males between 18 and 35 who live in the greater San Diego, California area.

Ha1: Self-efficacy in terms of using condoms and self-perceived susceptibility to HIV/AIDS adequately predict, individually or in linear combination, self-reported likelihood of condom use among African American males between 18 and 35 who live in the greater San Diego, California area.

Threats to Validity

External Validity

To mitigate biased responding, anonymity was provided to study participants. Each participant was reminded of the anonymous nature of the study and the importance of honest responses to survey questions. The study design did not

restrict the user from completing multiple surveys or ensuring that one individual completes the survey without another person's influence; however, participants were reminded that they can only participate in the study once and they should be the only one to respond to the items. A filter question to ensure that the participant has not completed the questionnaire previously was also added to the consent form to prevent participants from completing the questionnaire multiple times.

The nature of social media as a recruitment vehicle was not without challenge; however, researchers have established the merits of its use as a recruitment method for studies with a health emphasis (Fenner et al., 2012). External validation addresses the ability to generalize data across a large population of the group under scrutiny at varying time points and geographic location (Lingsma et al., 2015).

Several different methods were used to recruit individuals from across the region in order to make the data as generalizable as possible. Although a convenience sampling technique has limited generalizability, the characteristics of the samples were compared to the population of African American males in San Diego, California to ensure that a representation was considered in the study. Data collection was focused on one specific population, and the findings will not be generalizable beyond that population.

Internal Validity

In correlation research, internal validation addresses the trustworthiness of the data. According to McGue et al (2010), threats to internal validity include the presence of confounding variables. The present study avoided this threat by focusing on specific predictor variables that represent the components of the HBM including self-efficacy, susceptibility, and health behavior. The use of valid and reliable methods also strengthens internal validity.

Ethical Procedures

The Institutional Review Board (IRB) provided approval for the study's use of human participants. No personally identifiable data was recorded from participants in order to ensure anonymity, and no IP addresses were collected. I aimed to conduct the study with high ethical standards. Participants were informed that no names or identifying information were collected. An informed consent informed participants about their right to withdraw at any time or refuse to participate. The participants first accessed the consent form and provide consent by clicking on the "I consent" button after which they will be able to access the survey questions. Once data was collected and downloaded, all survey information was permanently removed from the Survey Monkey site.

All data was stored in a password-protected computer only accessible to the researcher and will be destroyed seven years after publication. In order to address any potential psychological distress, a link was provided to access a counseling hotline and a resource link to health testing centers so that individuals who are concerned that they may be at risk of having contracted a sexually transmitted disease can seek testing and treatment.

Summary

The research design was quantitative in nature and designed to measure predictive relationships between self-perceived susceptibility and self-efficacy (independent variables), and condom use (the dependent variable). A sample of 18- to 35- year-old African American men from San Diego, CA was used. Ordinal logistic regression was originally planned for analysis; however, I used binary logistic regression to determine if there was any predictive relationship between independent variables and the dependent variable.

Questionnaires were used to assess independent variables, and the dependent variable was assessed using a nominal scale.

The HBM was used to guide the study. External validity was supported through selection of participants. Participants were anonymous.

CHAPTER 4: Results

Introduction

The purpose of this quantitative survey study was to examine the extent to which self-efficacy and self-perceived susceptibility to HIV/AIDS predict self-reported likelihood of condom use during sexual activities among African American males who reside in San Diego, CA. The population of 18- to 35-year-old African American men living in California is uniquely at risk to contract HIV/AIDS (Funk et al., 2018).

These men have a greater incidence of delayed treatment and diagnosis for HIV/AIDS compared to their Caucasian counterparts (Henny et al., 2012). Low-income status, unemployment, incarceration, and low education disproportionately impact this population, all of which are factors that are also associated with increased rates of HIV/AIDS infection (Henny et al., 2012; Millett et al., 2012).

It is not known if and to what extent self-efficacy and self-perceived susceptibility to HIV/AIDS predict self- reported likelihood of condom use during sexual activities among African American males living in San Diego, CA.

Condom use was studied as a variable based on its documented effectiveness in terms of preventing HIV/AIDS infection.

Encouraging consistent use of condoms is a predictor of positive health outcomes which leads to reduced incidence of HIV/AIDS diagnosis among African American males (Shepherd et al., 2014). Self-perceived susceptibility and perceived self-efficacy were used as predictor variables while self- reported likelihood of condom use during sexual activity was measured as the dependent variable. A binary logistic regression was conducted to determine if self-perceived susceptibility and perceived self-efficacy were significant predictors of condom use during sexual activity.

A single research question was analyzed in the study:

RQ1: Do self-efficacy in terms of using condoms and self-perceived susceptibility to HIV/AIDS adequately predict, individually or in linear combination, self-reported likelihood of condom use among African American males between 18 and 35 who live in the greater San Diego, California area?

H01: Self-efficacy in terms of using condoms and self-perceived susceptibility to HIV/AIDS do not adequately predict, individually or in linear combination, self-reported likelihood of condom use among African American males between 18 and 35 who live in the greater San Diego, California area.

Ha1: Self-efficacy in terms of using condoms and self-perceived susceptibility to HIV/AIDS adequately predict, individually or in linear combination, self-reported likelihood of condom use among African American males between 18 and 35 who live in the greater San Diego, California area.

In this chapter, I describe the data collection, including response rates. I also discuss characteristics of the sample, including demographic information and statistics involving condom use and health status information. I also report results of analyses that were used to test hypotheses. Finally, I provide a chapter summary.

Data Collection

A convenience sample of 18 to 35-year-old African American men was recruited following the plan as explained in Chapter 3, with some limitations given the COVID-19 pandemic.

African American churches as well as alumni associations of historically Black colleges and universities in the San Diego, CA area were contacted with invitations to take part in this research. Participants were recruited within a 26-mile radius of the city center of San Diego.

The original recruitment strategy was to use San Diego-based barbers who would post flyers in high traffic areas. Barbershops are an important institution in the African American community where men gather to discuss important topics while waiting for services (Cottrell & McKenzie, 2011; Warren-Findlow et al., 2012).

However, traditional methods of outreach and recruitment were hindered due to social distancing requirements of the 2019 COVID-19 pandemic. Barbershop closures due to COVID-19 mandates hindered my ability to obtain many recruits within the barbershop community initially, but as COVID-19 restrictions were eased, recruitment through barbershops increased.

In response to barriers for recruitment, Facebook and other social media platforms promoting local African American themed clubs and organizations throughout the San Diego area were added as targeted areas for recruitment following IRB approval (see Appendix G). Sample size was calculated using G*Power v3.1.0 and a minimum sample of 113 participants was calculated and recruited for the purpose of screening a representative sample.

Response Rates

Data collection began on February 1, 2021 and ended on May 13, 2021. A total of 145 participants responded to the survey.

Seventy-two percent of these participants completed the entire questionnaire, resulting in 105 completed surveys, which left the study slightly underpowered. There were no consistent patterns that were observed among those who did not complete the study. Some participants discontinued during the middle of the survey, while other participants discontinued three quarters into the survey. Premature discontinuation may be attributable to the length of the survey. According to Le et al. (2021), survey fatigue is a phenomenon in which respondents become tired, bored, and uninterested in surveys.

Due to the nature of the study, respondents were at risk of becoming fatigued, and completion rates were negatively impacted by this phenomenon. Only respondents who completed the entire survey were included in the final analysis.

Chi-square tests of independence were conducted on demographic variables to determine if there were statistically significant differences between those who completed the survey and those who did not. Results indicated that there were no significant differences between those who completed the study and those who did not in terms of highest level of education completed ($\chi2$ (4, n = 145) = .354, p = .99), sexual orientation ($\chi2$ (3, n = 145) = .289, p = .96), number of sexual partners ($\chi2$ (5, n = 145) = .081, p = 1.0), and frequency of sexual activity ($\chi2$ (2, n = 145) = .159, p = .92). These results suggested that study completers and non-completers were similar, and those included in the final database were likely not a select group of individuals.

Characteristics of the Sample

African American male populations in the U.S. have been reported to experience increased susceptibility to HIV/AIDS and other STDs in comparison to other ethnic groups (Lyles et al., 2007). Further understanding of the mechanisms of disease prevention can impact health outcomes for this population.

As Montanaro and Bryan (2014) have suggested, the Health Belief Model and the Theory of Planned Behavior (TPB) predict and can influence change in health behaviors. Bandura (1978) said a person's actions are influenced by perceptions of individual levels of self-efficacy.

The sample was recruited by placing flyers and posters at specific venues using venue-based sampling and targeting predominantly African American churches, barber shops, and historically Black colleges and universities alumni groups located in San Diego, CA (Cottrell & McKenzie, 2011; Warren-Findlow, 2012).

A total of 105 African American male respondents completed the study. Of those, 51.4% had not graduated high school, had a high school diploma, or a GED. Over 90% identified as heterosexual and 21.9% reported having an STD at some time in their life. Of respondents, 62.9% indicated they used condoms at least most of the time. Finally, condom use self-efficacy had a mean of 114.79 (SD = 15.73), where higher scores represented higher self-efficacy. According to the USCB (2017b), there are 47,380 African American men in San Diego County, CA.

Therefore, the sample size of 105 constituted 1/1000 of a percent of the total population. Given this small proportion and that a convenience sampling approach was used, the sample may not be representative of the larger population. This was a limitation of the study (see Table 1).

Table 1
Characteristics of Participants

	N	%	Mean	SD
Age	105		26.34	4.29
Education				
Less than a high school degree	3	2.9		
High school graduate or GED	51	48.6		
Associates degree	20	19.0		
Bachelor's degree	27	25.7		
Advanced degree	5	3.8		
Sexual orientation				
Heterosexual	99	94.3		
Gay	2	1.9		
Bisexual	3	2.9		
Other	1	1.0		
Diagnosed STDs				
Chlamydia	19	18.1		
Herpes	2	1.9		
Trichomoniasis	2	1.9		
Gonorrhea	3	2.9		
NGU/NSU	1	1.0		
HIV	1	1.0		
Genital warts	1	1.0		
Syphilis	0	0.0		
None of the above	26	24.8		
No previous diagnoses	49	46.7		
Condom use (with new or non-steady partners)				
Always	38	36.2		
Most of the time	28	26.7		
Sometimes	21	20.0		
Rarely	6	5.7		
Never	12	11.4		
Visited clinic because concerned about risk for STD/HIV				
Yes	22	21.0		
No	83	79.0		

Due to rounding, percentages may not add up to 100

Results

There are three phases in the data analysis process. The first phase is the data preparation phase. During this phase, the data is first checked for missing data and data errors. As stated above, there were 40 participants with incomplete data who were removed from the database. There were no data errors detected. Also, during this phase, new variables are computed, if necessary, and composite scores are created. Condom Self-Efficacy composite scores were computed, where the scores for all 26 questions were summed together to compute a composite total score. Additionally, Perceived Risk of HIV was dummy coded, based on responses, where 1 was at risk and 0 was not at risk.

This computation was used because only one question reflected HIV risk, "What was the reason for visiting an STD clinic, do you think you could be at risk for an STD/HIV?" where 1 was yes and 0 was no. Finally, condom usage was also dummy coded as 0, inconsistent condom usage (never, rarely, sometimes, most of the time), and 1, consistent condom usage (always).

According to Hounton et al. (2005) previous studies have used the Likert Scale as a measure of condom use in men. A dummy coded scale was used because the sample size across two of the four choices was 12 or less. This was not large enough to conduct an ordinal regression (Tabachnick & Fidell, 2013). Therefore, a binomial logistic regression was utilized.

The second phase was the preliminary analysis phase. This phase consisted of checking the assumptions of the binomial regression including: 1) the assumption of no multicollinearity, 2) the outcome variable is dichotomous, and 3) the predictor variables are categorical and/or continuous (Field, 2018; Pallant, 2020). The assumptions for the outcome variable were met as the variable was scored on a 0 and 1 dichotomous scale. The assumption of the predictor variables was met, as Condom Use Self-Efficacy was a continuous variable and Perceived Risk was a dichotomous variable.

Additionally, no evidence of multicollinearity between predictors variables was found, as the Variance Inflation Factor (VIF) was below 5 (tolerance = .999, VIF = 1.001). The assumption of independent observations was also met because cases were independent of each other. Finally, the assumption of large sample size was also met, as the sample size is above 30 (Field, 2018; Pallant, 2020).

The third and final phase of the data analysis process is the primary analysis phase. During this phase, the null hypothesis of the research question is tested. To address the research question, a binomial logistic regression was conducted. The binomial logistic regression is conducted when you want to predict the outcome of a dichotomous outcome variable, by one or more continuous and categorical predictor variables.

In this study there were two predictor variables and one outcome variable. The first predictor variable was the CUSES score (Brafford & Beck, 1991). The Likert scale scores ranged from 1 to 5 where 1 was strongly agree, and 5 was strongly disagree. The second predictor variable was Perceived Risk of HIV (Hounton et al., 2005), where 0, no perceived risk of HIV, and 1 was perceived risk of HIV. The outcome variable was Condom Use During Sex, where 1 was consistent condom use and 0 was inconsistent condom use.

The results of the binomial logistic regression indicated that the model was significant predictor for always using condoms among African American men ($\chi 2 = 18.12$, $p < .001$), where the model explained 15.9% (Cox & Snell R) to 21.7% (Nagelkerke R) of the variability in condom use score. The model accurately predicted 75.2% of the cases, compared to 63.8% accuracy in the baseline model.

A review of the coefficients table indicated that Condom Use Self-Efficacy made a significant contribution to the model (Exp () = 1.06, $p < .001$), where a unit increase in Condom Self-Efficacy scores was associated with 1.06 time increase in the likelihood of using condoms consistently. Perceived Risk did not make a significant contribution to the model (Exp () = .39, $p = .11$). As a result of the logistic regression, the null hypothesis was rejected. (See Table 2)

Table 2
Binary Logistic Regression for Condom Use

	β	S.E.	Wald	df	Sig.	Exp(β)	95% C.I.for EXP(β) Lower	Upper
CUSES score	.058	.016	13.000	1	.000	1.059	1.027	1.093
Perceived Risk score	-.939	.587	2.563	1	.109	.391	.124	1.235
Constant	-7.110	1.894	14.095	1	.000	.001		

a. Variable(s) entered on step 1: CUSES score, Perceived Risk.

Summary

The purpose of this study was to determine if self-efficacy in terms of using condoms and self-perceived susceptibility to HIV/AIDS adequately predicted, individually or in linear combination, self-reported likelihood of condom use among African American males between 18- and 35 who live in the greater San Diego, CA. Results of this study indicated that this was a significant predictor of condom use among African American men, improving prediction accuracy over the baseline model by 11.4%. Perceived risk did not significantly contribute to the model. However, condom use self-efficacy contributed to the model where a unit increase in condom self-efficacy scores was associated with 1.06 times increase in the likelihood of using condoms consistently.

Chapter 5 includes a discussion of results. Results were discussed in the context of the literature review. Specifically, Chapter 5 includes results of this as well as previous similar studies. Chapter 5 includes interpretations and analysis of findings along with recommendations for future research based on limitations of the current study.

CHAPTER 5: Discussion, Conclusions, And Recommendations

Introduction

The objective of this quantitative survey study was to examine the extent to which self-efficacy and self-perceived susceptibility to HIV/AIDS predict self-reported likelihood of condom use during sexual activities among African American males who reside in San Diego County, CA. The population of 18–35-year-old African American men living in California are at high risk of contracting HIV/AIDS (Funk et al., 2018). In addition to increased risk of STI, a larger proportion of these men receive delayed diagnosis and treatment for HIV/AIDS than their Caucasian counterparts (Henny et al., 2012). Given how damaging delayed diagnosis and treatment of HIV/AIDS can be, promoting condom use among African American males to reduce HIV/AIDS infection may be a viable remedy to these issues. As a result, research examining the extent to which self-efficacy and self-perceived susceptibility to HIV/AIDS predicts self-reported likelihood of condom use during sexual activities is critically important.

I examined if self-efficacy in terms of using condoms and self-perceived susceptibility to HIV/AIDS predicted, individually or in combination, condom use as reported by the population of interest, which was African American males who were between 18 and 35 living in the greater San Diego area. A binomial logistic regression analysis was conducted to address the research question. Predictor variables were self-efficacy in terms of using condoms and self-perceived susceptibility to HIV/AIDS. The outcome variable was self-reported condom use.

Results indicated that the model was significant, where the model explained 15.9% (Cox & Snell R) to 21.7% (Nagelkerke R) of the variability in condom use scores.

Specifically, a unit increase in condom self-efficacy scores was associated with 1.06 time increase in the likelihood of using condoms consistently. Perceived risk did not make contribute to the model. As a result of the logistic regression analysis, the null hypothesis was rejected.

Interpretation of Findings

Theoretical Model

Bandura (1978) said a person's actions are influenced by perceptions of their level of self-efficacy. According to Bandura (1978), people's beliefs in their own ability to create an expected outcome directly relates to the likelihood of taking actions that will lead to productive outcomes. Based on Bandura's SLT, it was expected that as self- efficacy involving use of condoms increased, the likelihood of using condoms would also increase. Statistical analyses indicated that results were consistent.

Specifically, higher condom use self-efficacy scores predicted consistent condom use.

The HBM involves identifying how individuals make decisions that influence their health (Conner & Norman, 2006). Individual attitudes and beliefs are important factors in terms of making decisions related to one's health. According to Lin et al. (2005), HBM explains and predicts risky behaviors that can lead to poor health outcomes, namely acquiring sexually transmitted infections resulting from unprotected sexual activity with an HIV/AIDS infected partner.

Their work is an example of the linkage specifically between perceived susceptibility and preventive health behavior. Based on the HBM, it was expected that perceived risk of HIV/AIDS would be a significant predictor of consistent condom use. In the current study, perceived risk of HIV/AIDS was not a significant predictor of consistent condom use. Therefore, results did not align with expected outcomes.

Key Literature Findings

Self-efficacy is defined as individual perceptions of ability to control surroundings to create behavioral changes and lead to positive health outcomes (Wideman et al., 2014). Alvy et al. (2011) said self-efficacy was instrumental in terms of improving depressed mood, overcoming addiction to smoking, and implementing consistent condom usage. Bauni and Jarabi (2003) said self-efficacy might influence the ability to overcome barriers to prevention strategies, which could improve health outcomes. The work of Bauni and Jarabi (2003) also suggests that the psychological influences at work in the prevention of sexually transmitted infections can be understood through the study of self-efficacy.

Based on findings in previous research, it was expected that self-efficacy would be related to consistent condom use. Specifically, increases in self-efficacy might be related to consistent condom use because higher values on the self-efficacy scale predicted a 1 on the consistent condom use scale. Results of the current study indicated that condom use self-efficacy made a significant contribution to the model.

Specifically, a unit increase in condom self-efficacy scores was associated with a 1.06 time increase in terms of likelihood of using condoms consistently. In summary, results aligned with expected findings, as evidenced by research in the literature review.

Maddux and Rogers (1983) said susceptibility to a known health risk can prompt behavior changes in order to deal with to health risks. Brooks et al. (2009) said perceived susceptibility to HIV/AIDS was positively associated with condom usage. Additionally, according to Maiman and Becker (1974), the greater a person's perceive susceptibility, the greater the threat perception, which may lead to taking decisive actions to minimize or eliminate the threat.

Results indicated that the model to predict consistent condom use was significant, but perceived risk did not make a significant contribution to the model. Therefore, results did not align entirely with previous findings related to perceived susceptibility as reported in the literature review. This may be because the scale for consistent condom use was changed for the analysis, with only two values. It may have resulted in less sensitivity to detect meaningful predictive relationships with condom use.

In this current study, self-perceived susceptibility to HIV/AIDS was evaluated as a variable using the Perceived Risk Scale. Based on research on perceived susceptibility in the literature review, it was expected that increases in self-perceived susceptibility to HIV/AIDS would be related to increases in terms of likelihood of using condoms.

However, this was not the case in the current study because the relationship was not linear, given that the dependent variable, consistent condom use, was coded 0 and 1.

Therefore, the relationship was based on likelihood of consistent condom use, as opposed to a linear relationship in previous research.

Limitations of the Study

One of the limitations of the study was the lower than targeted sample size of 113 participants. A total of 145 participants responded to the survey. Seventy-two percent of these participants completed the entire questionnaire, resulting in 105 completed surveys, which left the study slightly underpowered. Post-hoc power analysis revealed the statistical power for the binomial logistic regression to be .39. The resultant power was lower than the .80 threshold that is considered acceptable in the social, business, and health sciences (Field, 2018; Pallant, 2020).

A power of .39 indicates that there is only a 39% chance of detecting a significant effect if one exists in the entire population. Given the low statistical power, there are constraints on implications of this study regarding positive social change and recommendations for practice.

As stated previously, the reported power of .39 is below the minimum standard of .80 or 80% likelihood of detecting a significant effect if one actually exists in the population. There were no consistent patterns observed among those who did not complete the study.

Only one of the two predictor variables was significant. This may be attributed to decreased statistical power with regards to the sample size. It may also be due to the dependent variable, consistent condom use, being coded as 1 and 0. This potentially led to lack of nuance in terms of relationships among variables due to not using the Likert scale for the dependent variable. However, the dichotomous transformation was required due to low sample sizes for some of the Likert items.

An additional limitation of the study was the convenience sampling approach. With convenience sampling, researchers accept respondents, anyone who is available and meets the selection criteria. The drawback regarding this sampling approach is that it may not produce a sample that is representative of the target population (Creswell, 2013; Leedy & Ormrod, 2018).

Therefore, the results of this study may not be generalizable to the larger target population. The benefit of the convenience sampling method is the assurance of survey participants.

Despite the hindrances of mandatory social isolation in response to a global pandemic, I was able to reach qualified participants in order to complete the desired research aims. In future studies, a larger sample size would be targeted to address the need for increased power within the sample and to overcome the challenge associated with survey fatigue amongst the participants.

Self-reported survey data was another limitation of the study, as it relied solely on memory, self-perception, and truthfulness of the respondents, is a potential limitation of the data (Creswell, 2013). This study was limited to identifying predictive relationships between variables, because the research design is not focused on identifying causation between variables. Therefore, in no way can the findings be used to conclude that the independent variables directly influence the dependent variable in a causal manner. The study is limited to determining whether self-efficacy and perceived susceptibility to HIV/AIDS infection predict consistent condom usage among African American males.

Recommendations

Several recommendations are established based on the results of this study. First, the sample size target of 113, which produces a statistical power of .80, appears not to be ideal for the purposes of repeating this study as 105 is not close to 113.

A larger sample size was needed to achieve adequate statistical power. Statistical power is the probability of a significant effect in calculated analysis if the effect exists in the entire population (Field, 2018; Pallant, 2020). Given that the sample size was below the target size and power, it may be that Perceived Risk of HIV/AIDS was not a significant predictor because of the smaller sample size. Although 145 participants began the surveys, it is important to possibly improve the instructions and potentially program a "percentage complete" monitor in the survey instrument to reduce the number of surveys that were incomplete.

As a result, it is recommended that future studies ensure that the target sample size for a statistical power of .80 is reached. Given the low power, it cannot be stated definitively that self-perceived susceptibility to HIV/AIDS does not have an effect on condom usage. According to previous literature, it can be surmised that the effect was not large enough in size to be detected as significant.

A second recommendation for this study is that it be conducted among African American men in other states, including northern, southern, and mid-western states. The slight historical and cultural differences that exist regionally may have an impact on African American males perceived self-efficacy and consistency in condom usage. However, given that condom use was coded as 1 used consistent condom use and 0 was coded for inconsistent condom use, degrees of condom usage were not captured.

Additionally, future research of this kind may find that condom use self-efficacy and self- perceived susceptibility may differ by region and state. Large metropolitan areas may have increased prevalence of HIV/AIDS interventions that promote increase perceived risk of HIV and increased condom usage self-efficacy in contrast to suburban and rural areas, where public health messaging may be less frequent.

However, the ability to assess this possibility was limited given the low sample size, and the dichotomous nature of perceived risk of HIV and condom usage. Additionally, because this was a predictive study, it can only be said that a change in one variable is associated with a change in another variable.

Additional future research recommendations include conducting qualitative research to obtain an in-depth understanding of African American men's perceptions around condom usage, condom use self-efficacy, and self-perceived susceptibility to HIV/AIDS. The current research study suggested that self-perceived susceptibility to HIV/AIDS had no effect on condom usage. Presently, it is not known whether this was due to low statistical power, or whether it is not a predictive factor among the entire population of African American men. A qualitative study design would help provide insight on whether there is a sense of susceptibility to HIV/AIDS among African American men, and how extensive this perception is.

Furthermore, a qualitative research design may offer theories on behavioral practices as well as perceived vulnerability through in-depth interviews and specialized qualitative research methods. One of the drawbacks of a qualitative study is that anonymity would be no longer possible.

Implications for Positive Social Change

Individual

The Condom Use Self-Efficacy (CUSES: Brafford & Beck.,1991) includes 26 items related to self-efficacy with regards to condom use. Higher scores indicate higher perception of condom use efficacy. Sample statements include: "I feel confident in my ability to use a condom correctly" and "I feel confident in my ability to suggest using condoms with a new partner." Condom Use Self-Efficacy scores were predictive of using condoms consistently. Therefore, the implication on the individual is that those who are comfortable and confident with using condoms may use condoms consistently. Consistent use of condoms will likely decrease the spread of HIV/AIDS and other sexually transmitted diseases among this target population.

Society

More consistent condom usage among African American men will likely decrease the spread of HIV/AIDS among this community. Ultimately, a decrease in the prevalence of this sexually transmitted disease, which disproportionately affects African American men, would produce a positive impact on society. Increased condom usage may result in the lower prevalence of HIV/AIDS and other opportunistic diseases associated with HIV/AIDS. This would result in a healthier population, less need for family and community members to care for sick individuals, and less its impact on the health care system, which in turn would decrease costs associated with HIV/AIDs care. Increased condom use self-efficacy may also reduce the spread of other sexually transmitted diseases.

Finally, from a public health policy perspective, if research shows that increased condom use efficacy increases the likelihood of condom usage, then increased public health funding might be instrumental in improving education for African American men on how to use condoms properly and effectively as well as access to free condoms.

Methodological/Theoretical/Empirical

The frameworks for this study Bandura's (1978) SLT and the HBM (Lin et al., 2005). According to the social learning theory, people's beliefs in their own ability to create an expected outcome directly relates to the likelihood of taking actions that will lead to productive outcomes. It was expected that as self-efficacy in one's use of condoms increased, the likelihood of using condoms consistently would also increase. The results of the current study support this theoretical model. The results add support to the expanded scope and reach of the social learning theory to include self-efficacy in condom usage and increased consistency in condom usage among African American men.

For the HBM, an individual's attitudes and beliefs are essential factors in making decisions related to one's health (Conner & Norman, 2006). It was expected that Perceived Risk of HIV/AIDS would be a significant predictor of consistent condom usage. In the current study, perceived risk of HIV/AIDS was not a significant predictor of consistent condom usage. Alternatively, the results did not align with expected HBM theories. Therefore, the current study did not provide support for the HBM ability to explain and predict risky behaviors that can lead to acquiring sexually transmitted infections resulting from unprotected sexual activity with an HIV/AIDS infected partner.

Practice

The results of the research indicated that condom use self efficacy was predictive of consistent condom usage. Therefore, interventions that promote improved condom use self-efficacy would likely be effective at improving consistent condom use among African American men. One such that program that has been used is the Popular Opinion Leader (POL) approach (Kerr et al., 2018). POL is an HIV prevention intervention that involves identifying, enlisting, and training key opinion leaders to encourage safer sexual norms and behaviors within their social networks through risk reduction conversations (Kerr et al., 2018). The CDC offers technical assistance in implementing POL interventions for interested organizations, effectively endorsing this health behavioral strategy (Kelly et al., 1991).

Currently, it cannot be established if creating trainings and or interventions that promote self-perceived susceptibility to HIV/AIDS would increase consistent condom usage among African American men. This is because there was no significant self- perceived susceptibility effect in this study.

So, the implication is that the focus of training should be on condom use self-efficacy and not on self-perceived susceptibility to HIV/AIDS.

Conclusion

The current study offers findings that support current theories fand offer novel findings with respect to African American men who experience increased risk of HIV/AIDS. The study added to the current literature by supporting Bandura's (1978) Social Learning Theory, which argues that increased self-efficacy should be related to an individual's ability to create behavioral changes that prompt positive health outcomes.

The research contributes to the HIV/AIDS intervention literature by showing that increased condom use self-efficacy predicted consistent condom usage. Furthermore, findings indicate that the HBM might not be an appropriate model for developing a conceptual understanding of its impact on consistent condom usage. This finding is not widely reported in the literature and is a significant future research point of discussion. Lastly, this study revealed that condom use training could impact consistent condom usage among African American men. This finding is an important addition to the HIV/AIDS intervention literature.

African American men have a greater incidence of delayed treatment and diagnosis for HIV/AIDS compared to their Caucasian counterparts (Henny et al., 2012). Several factors such as low-income status, unemployment, incarceration, and low education disproportionately impact this population and are associated with increased HIV/AIDS infection (Henny et al., 2012; Millett et al., 2012).

The current study offers evidence that self-efficacy, but not self-perceived susceptibility to HIV/AIDS, predicts the self-reported likelihood of consistent condom use during sexual activities among African American males living in the San Diego area in California. There needs to be greater clarification as to whether self-perceived susceptibility to HIV/AIDS can have a positive impact on condom usage. Further exploration of this research question can be performed qualitatively. Additional improvements may be obtained by ensuring adequate samples population size to establish a statistical power that is relevant for statistical significance.

REFERENCES

Alvy, L. M., McKirnan, D. J., Mansergh, G., Koblin, B., Colfax, G. N., Flores S. A., Hudson, S., & Project MIX Study Group. (2011). Depression is associated with sexual risk among men who have sex with men but is mediated by cognitive escape and self-efficacy. AIDS and Behavior, 15(6),1171–1179.

Argüello, T. M., & Walters, K. (2018). They tell us "we don't belong in the world and we shouldn't take up a place": HIV discourse within two-spirit communities. *Journal of Ethnic & Cultural Diversity in Social Work, 27*(2), 107–123.

Baden, R., & Dolin, R. (2012). The road to an effective HIV vaccine. *New England Journal of Medicine, 366*(14), 1343–1344. https://www.nejm.org/doi/full/10.1056/NEJMe1202492

Bandura, A. (1978). Social learning theory of aggression. *Journal of Communication, 28*(3), 12–29.

Bauni, E. K., & Jarabi, B. O. (2003). The low acceptability and use of condoms within marriage: Evidence from Nakuru district, Kenya. *African Population Studies, 18*, 51–55.

Beyer, C., & Havlir, D. (2012). The beginning of the end of AIDS? *New England Journal of Medicine, 365*, 385–387. https://www.nejm.org/doi/10.1056/NEJMp1207138

Blanton, H., Gerrard, M., & McClive-Reed, K. P. (2013). Threading the needle in health- risk communication: Increasing vulnerability salience while promoting self-worth. *Journal of Health Communication*, *18*(11), 1279–1292.

Brafford, L. J., & Beck, K. H. (1991). Development and validation of a condom self- efficacy scale for college students. *Journal of American College Health*, *39*(5), 219-225.

Brooks, R. A., Lee, S. J., Stover, G. N., & Barkley, T. W., Jr. (2009). Condom attitudes, perceived vulnerability, and sexual risk behaviors of young Latino male urban street gang members: Implications for HIV prevention. *AIDS Education and Prevention: Official Publication of the International Society for AIDS Education*, *21*(suppl. B), 80–87.

Brown, L. K., & Lourie, K. J. (2000). Children and adolescents living with HIV and AIDS: A review. *Journal of Child Psychology and Psychiatry*, *41*(1), 81–96.

Brown, L., Lourie, K., & Pao, M. (2005). Children and adolescents living with HIV and AIDS: A review. *Journal of Child Psychology and Psychiatry and Allied Disciplines, 41*(1), 81–96. http://www.ncbi.nlm.nih.gov/pubmed/10763677

Campbell, A. N., Brooks, A. J., Pavlicova, M., Hu, M. C., Hatch-Maillette, M. A., Calsyn, D. A., & Tross, S. (2016).

Barriers to condom use: Results for men and women enrolled in HIV risk reduction trials in outpatient drug treatment. *Journal of HIV/AIDS & Social Services*, *15*(2), 130–146.

Campbell, D. T., & Stanley, J. C. (2015). *Experimental and quasi-experimental designs for research*. Ravenio Books.

Centers for Disease Control and Prevention. (2005). Antiretroviral postexposure prophylaxis after sexual, injection-drug use, or other nonoccupational exposure to HIV in the U.S.: Recommendations from the U.S. Department of Health and Human Services. *Morbidity and Mortality Weekly Report,54*(RR-2). http://www.cdc.gov/mmwr/PDF/rr/rr5402.pdf

Chomsky, N. (1959). A review of BF Skinner's *Verbal Behavior*. *Language*, *35*(1), 26– 58.

Clement, S., Schauman, O., Graham, T., Maggioni, F., Evans-Lacko, S., Bezborodovs, N., Morgan, C., Rüsch, N., Brown, J. S. L., & Thornicroft, G. (2015). What is the impact of mental health-related stigma on help-seeking? A systematic review of quantitative and qualitative studies. *Psychological Medicine, 45*(1), 11–27.

Coates, T. J. (1990). Strategies for modifying sexual behavior for primary and secondary prevention of HIV disease. *Journal of Consulting and Clinical Psychology, 58*(1), 57. https://doi.org/10.1037/0022-006X.58.1.57

Colbert, J. (2012). Preexposure prophylaxis for HIV prevention—Polling results. *New England Journal of*

Medicine, 367, e22. https://www.nejm.org/doi/full/10.1056/NEJMclde1211517

Conner, M., & Norman, P. (Eds.). (2006). *Predicting health behavior*. Open University Press & McGraw-Hill Education.

Cottrell, R. R., & McKenzie, J. (2011). *Health promotion and education research methods: Using the five-chapter thesis/dissertation model* (2nd ed.). Jones & Bartlett Publishers.

Creswell, J. W. (2013). Qualitative inquiry: Choosing among five approaches (3rd ed.).SAGE Publications.

Crosby, R., Salazar, L. F., & DiClemente, J. (2014). Lack ofrecent condom use among detained adolescent males: A multilevel investigation. *Sexually Transmitted Infections, 80*(6). https://sti.bmj.com/content/80/6/425

Crosby, R. A., Milhausen, R. R., Graham, C. A., Yarber, W. L., Sanders, S. A., Charnigo, R., & Shrier, L. A. (2014). Likelihood of condom use when sexually transmitted diseases are suspected. *Health Education & Behavior, 41*(4), 449–454. https://doi.org/10.1177/1090198114529588

Davis, K. R., & Weller, S. C. (1999). The effectiveness of condoms in reducing heterosexual transmission of HIV. *Family Planning Perspectives*, 272–279. https://www.guttmacher.org/pubs/journals/3127299.html

Deeks, S. G., Lewin, S. R., & Havlir, D. V. (2013). The

end of AIDS: HIV infection as a chronic disease. *The Lancet, 382*(9903), 1525–1533. https://doi.org/10.1016/S0140-6736(13)61809-7

DiClemente, R. J., Wingood, G. M., Harrington, K. F., Lang, D. L., Davies, S. L., Hook, E. W., III, Oh, M. K., Crosby, R. A., Hertzberg, V. S.,Gordon, A. B., Hardin, J. W., Parker, S., & Robillard, A. (2004). Efficacy of an HIV prevention intervention for AfricanAmerican adolescent girls: A randomized controlled trial. *The Journal of the American Medical Association, 292*(2), 171–179.

Fauci, A. S. (2012). Toward an AIDS-free generation. *The Journal of the American Medical Association 308*(4), 343–368. https://doi.org/10.1001/jama.2012.8142

Fenner, Y., Garland, S. M., Moore, E. E., Jayasinghe, Y., Fletcher, A., Tabrizi, S. N., Gunasekaran, B., & Wark, J. D. (2012). Web-based recruiting for health research using a social networking site: An exploratory study. *Journal of Medical Internet Research*, *14*(1).

Field, A. P. (2018). *Discovering statistics using IBM SPSS statistics* (5th ed.). SAGE Publishing.

Fisher, J. D., & Fisher, W. A. (2000). Theoretical approaches to individual-level change in HIV risk behavior. In *Handbook of HIV prevention* (pp. 3–55). Springer US.

Fisher, B., Sallis, J., & Neville, O. (2008). Ecological models of health behavior. In K. Glanz, B. K. Rimer, & K. Viswanath

(Eds.), *Health behavior and health education: Theory, research, and practice* (pp. 465–485). Jossey-Bass.

Forsyth, A. D., Carey, M. P., & Fuqua, R. W. (1997). Evaluation of the validity of the Condom Use Self-Efficacy Scale (CUSES) in young men using two behavioral simulations. *Health Psychology*, *16*(2), 175.

French, S. E., & Holland, K. J. (2013). Condom negotiation strategies as a mediator of the relationship between self-efficacy and condom use. *Journal of Sex Research*, *50*(1), 48–59. https://doi.org/10.1080/00224499.2011.626907

Funk, A. N., Inungu, J. N., Leveille, E. R., & Minelli, M. (2018). Factors associated with HIV-testing among African Americans: Analysis of the 2016 National Health Interview Survey. *European Journal of Environment and Public Health, 2*(1), 3.

Gerrard, M., Gibbons, F. X., & Bushman, B. J. (1996). Relation between perceived susceptibility to HIV and precautionary sexual behavior. *Psychological Bulletin, 119*(3), 390.

Graham, J. D., & Bray, S. R. (2015). Self-control strength depletion reduces self-efficacy and impairs exercise performance. *Journal of Sport & Exercise Psychology, 37*(5), 477–488.

Grusec, J. E. (1992). Social learning theory and developmental psychology: The legacies of Robert Sears and Albert Bandura. *Developmental Psychology, 28*(5), 776.

Gulette, D. L., Wright, P. B., Booth, B. M., Feldman, Z., & Stewart, K. E. (2009). Stages of change, decisional balance, and self-efficacy in condom use among rural African American stimulant users. *Journal of the Association of Nurses in AIDS Care, 20*(6), 428–441.

Henny, K. D., Crepaz, N., Lyles, C. M., Marshall, K. J., Aupont, L. W., Jacobs, E. D., Liau, A., Rama, S., Kay, L. S., Willis, L. A., & Charania, M. R. (2012). Efficacy of HIV/STI behavioral interventions for heterosexual African American men in the United States:A meta-analysis. *AIDS and Behavior, 16*(5), 1092–1114.

Hochbaum, G., Kegels, S., & Rosenstock, I. (1952). *Health belief model.* United States Public Health Service. Hounton, S. H., Carabin, H., & Henderson, N. J. (2005). Towards an understanding of barriers to condom use in rural Benin using the health belief model: A cross sectional survey. *BMC Public Health*, *5*(1), 1.

Houlding, C., & Davidson, R. (2003). Beliefs as predictors of condom use by injecting drug users in treatment. *Health Education Research*, *18*(2), 145–155.

Jemmott, L. S., Jemmott, J. B., Lanier, Y., Thompson, C., & Baker, J. L. (2017). Development of a barbershop-based HIV/STI risk reduction intervention for young heterosexual African American men. *Health Promotion Practice*, *18*(1), 110–118.

Johnson, V. A., Calvez, V., Gunthard, H. F., Paredes, R., Pillay, D., Shafer, R. W., Wensing, A. M., & Richman, D. D.

(2013). Update of the drug resistance mutations in HIV-1: March 2013. *Topics in Antiviral Medicine, 21*(1), 6–14.

Jones, C. L., Jensen, J. D., Scherr, C. L., Brown, N. R., Christy, K., & Weaver, J. (2015). The health belief model as an explanatory framework in communication research: Exploring parallel, serial, and moderated mediation. *Health Communication, 30*(6), 566–576.

Karim, S. S. A., Gray, G. E., & Martinson, N. (2012). Preexposure prophylaxis for HIV prevention. *The New England Journal of Medicine, 367*(5), 462–465. https://doi.org/10.1056/NEJMclde1207706

Kaufman, M. R., Rimal, R. N., Carrasco, M., Fajobi, O., Soko, A., Limaye, R., & Mkandawire, G. (2014). Using social and behavior change communication to increase HIV testing and condom use: The Malawi BRIDGE Project. *AIDS Care, 26*(supplement 1), S46–S49.

Kennedy, S. B., Nolen, S., Applewhite, J., Pan, Z., Shamblen, S., & Vanderhoff, K. J. (2007). A quantitative study on the condom-use behaviors of eighteen- to twenty- four-year- old urban African American males. *AIDS Patient Care and STDS, 21*(5), 306–320. https://doi.org/10.1089/apc.2006.0105

Kerr, Z. Y., Register-Mihalik, J. K., Haarbauer-Krupa, J., Kroshus, E., Go, V., Gildner, P., Byrd, K. H., & Marshall, S. W. (2018). Using opinion leaders to address intervention gaps in concussion prevention in youth sports: Key concepts and foundational theory. *Injury Epidemiology, 5*(28). https://doi.org/10.1186/s40621-018-0158-7

Laerd Statistics. (2018). *Ordinal regression using SPSS Statistics*.https://statistics.laerd.com/spstutorials/ordinalregression-using-spssstatistics.php

Laurencin, C. T., Christensen, D. M., & Taylor, E. D. (2008). HIV/AIDS and the African American community: A state of emergency. *Journal of the National Medical Association, 100*(1), 35–43.

Le, A., Han, B. H., & Palamar, J. J. (2021). When national drug surveys "take too long": An examination of who is at risk for survey fatigue. *Drug and alcohol dependence*, *225*, 108769.

Leedy, P. D., & Ormrod, J. E. (2015). Practical research. Planning and design (11th ed.). Boston, MA: Pearson

Letvin, N. L., Barouch, D. H., & Montefiori, D. C. (2002). Prospects for vaccine protection against HIV-1 infection and AIDS. *Annual Review of Immunology,* 20(1), 73–99.

Lifshitz, R., Nimrod, G., & Bachner, Y. G. (2016). Measuring risk perception in later life: The perceived risk scale. *Journal of the American Psychiatric Nurses Association, 22*(6), 469–474. https://doi.org/10.1177/1078390316659910

Lin, P., Simoni, J., & Zemon, V. (2005). The health belief model, sexual behaviors, and HIV risk among Taiwanese immigrants. *AIDS Education and Prevention, 17*(5), 469–483. https://doi.org/10.1521/aeap.2005.17.5.469

Lingsma, H. F., Yue, J. K., Maas, A. I. R., Steyerberg, E. W., Manley, G. T., Cooper, S. R., Dams-O'Connor, K., Gordon, W. A., Menon, D. K., Mukherjee, P., Okonkwo D. O., Puccio, A. M., Schnyer, D. M., Valadka, A. B., Vassar, M. J., & Yuh, E. L. (2015). Outcome prediction after mild and complicated mild traumatic brain injury: External validation of existing models and identification of new predictors using the TRACK-TBI pilot study. *Journal of Neurotrauma, 32*(2), 83–94

Loutfy, M. R., Sherr, L., Sonnenberg-Schwan, U., Walmsley, S. L., Johnson, M., & d'Arminio Monforte, A.. (2013). Caring for women living with HIV: Gaps in the evidence. *Journal of the International AIDS Society, 16*(1), 18509. https://doi.org/10.7448/IAS.16.1.18509

Lyles, C. M., Kay, L. S., Crepaz, N., Herbst, J. H., Passin, W. F., Kim, A. S., Rama, S. M., Thadiparthi, S., DeLuca, J. B., Mullins, M. M., & HIV/AIDS Prevention Research Synthesis Team. (2007). Best-evidence interventions: Findings from a systematic review of HIV behavioral interventions for US populations at high risk, 2000–2004. *American Journal of Public Health, 97*(1), 133–143.

Maddux, J. E., & Rogers, R. W. (1983). Protection motivation and self-efficacy: A revised theory of fear appeals and attitude change. *Journal of Experimental Social Psychology, 19*(5), 469–479: http://dx.doi.org/10.1016/0022-1031(83)90023-9

Maiman, L. A., & Becker, M. H. (1974). The health belief model: Origins and correlates in psychological theory. *Health Education Monographs*, *2*(4), 336–353. https://doi.org/10.1177/109019817400200404

Marriner, T. A., & Ralie, A. M. (2005). *Nursing theorists and their work* (5th ed.). Mason, M. J., Tanner, J. F., Piacentini, M., Freeman, D., Anastasia, T., Batat, W., Boland, W., Canbulut, M., Drenten, J., Hamby, A., Rangan, P., & Yang, Z., (2013). Advancing a participatory approach for youth risk behavior: Foundations, distinctions, and research directions. *Journal of Business Research,* 66(8), 1235–1241.

McCullagh, P. (1980). Regression models for ordinal data. *Journal of the Royal Statistical Society*: *Series B (Methodological), 42*(2), 109–127.

McGue, M., Osler, M., & Christensen, K. (2010). Causal inference and observational research: The utility of twins. *Perspectives on Psychological Science*, *5*(5), 546– 556.

Millett, G. A., Peterson, J. L., Flores, S. A., Hart, T. A., Jeffries, W. L., IV, Wilson, P. A.,Rourke, S. B., Heilig, C. M., Elford, J., Fenton, K. A., & Remis, R. S. (2012). Comparisons of disparities and risks of HIV infection in Black and other men who have sex with men in Canada, UK, and USA: A meta-analysis. *The Lancet, 380*(9839), 341–348.

Montanaro, E. A., & Bryan, A. D. (2014). Comparing theory-based condom interventions: Health belief model versus theory of planned behavior. *Health Psychology*, *33*(10), 1251.

Mustanski, B., Starks, T., & Newcomb, M. E. (2014). Methods for the design and analysis of relationship and partner effects on sexual health. *Archives of Sexual Behavior*, *43*(1), 21–33. https://doi.org/10.1007/s10508-013-0215-9

Nash, J. C. (2008). Re-thinking intersectionality. *Feminist Review, 89,* 1–15.
Streeck, H & Nixon, D. E.(2010). T cell immunity in acut HIV-1 infection. *Journal of Infectious Diseases*, *202*(supplement 2), S302-S308.https://pubmed.ncbi.nlm.nih.gov/20846037/

National Association of Social Workers. (2005). *HIV/AIDS and adolescents and young adults. A fact sheet for practitioners.* http://www.naswdc.org/practice/hiv_aids/ hiv_factsheet.asp

Nunn, A., Cornwall, A., Chute, N., Sanders, J., Thomas, G., James, G., Lally, M., Trooskin, S., & Flanigan, T. (2012). Keeping the faith: African American faith leaders' perspectives and recommendations for reducing racial disparities in HIV/AIDS infection. *PLoS One*, *7*(5), e36172.

Pallant, J. (2020). Factor analysis. In *SPSS survival manual* (7th ed.). McGraw-Hill. Pappas, S. (2012, February 26). *Condom uses 101: Basic errors are so common, study finds.* NBC News. https://www.nbcnews.com/healthmain/condom-use-101-basicerrors-are-so-common-study-finds-207925

Perepiczka, M., Chandler, N., & Becerra, M. (2011).
Relationship between graduate students' statistics selfefficacy, statistics anxiety, attitude toward statistics, and social support. *The Professional Counselor: Research and Practice,1*(2), 99–108.

Protogerou, C., & Hagger, M. S. (2016). Developing an integrated theoretical model of young peoples' condom use in sub-Saharan Africa. *Australian Journal of Psychology, 69*(2).

Quinn, T. C. (2002). The global HIV/AIDS pandemic 2002: A status report. *The Hopkins HIV Report,* 14(5), 12–15.

Reid, A. E., Dovidio, J. F., Ballester, E., & Johnson, B. T. (2014). HIV prevention interventions to reduce sexual risk for African Americans: The influence of community-level stigma and psychological processes. *Social Science & Medicine*, *103*,118–125.

Rhodes, S. D., Alonzo, J., Mann, L., Song, E. Y., Tanner, A. E., Arellano, J. E., Rodriguez-Celedon, R., Garcia, M., Freeman, A., Reboussin, B. A., & Painter, T. M. (2017). Small-group randomized controlled trial to increase condom use and HIV testing among Hispanic/Latino gay, bisexual, and other men who have sex with men. *American Journal of Public Health*, *107*(6), 969–976. https://doi.org/10.2105/AJPH.2017.303814

Schwarzer, R., & Luszczynska, A. (2011). Health behavior constructs: Theory, measurement, & research. *Self-Efficacy*.

http://cancercontrol.cancer.gov/brp/constructs/self-efficacy/se2.html

Shepherd, J., Harden, A., Barnett-Page, E., Kavanagh, J., Picot, J., Frampton, G. K., Cooper, K., Hartwell, D., & Clegg, A. (2014). Using process data to understand outcomes in sexual health promotion: An example from a review of schoolbased programs to prevent sexually transmitted infections. *Health Education Research, 29*(4), 566–582.

Stein, R., Song, W., Marano, M., Patel, H., Rao, S., &Morris, E. (2017). HIV testing, linkage to HIV medical care, and interviews for partner services among youths— 61 health department jurisdictions, United States, Puerto Rico, and the U.S. Virgin Islands, 2015. *Morbidity and Mortality Weekly Report*, *66*(24), 629.

Sutton, M. Y., & Parks, C. P. (2013). HIV/AIDS prevention, faith, and spirituality among Black/African American and Latino communities in the United States: Strengthening scientific faith-based efforts to shift the course of the epidemic and reduce HIV-related health disparities. *Journal of Religion and Health,* 52(2), 514– 530.

Sweeney, P., Gardner, L. I., Buchacz, K., Garland, P. M., Mugavero, M. J., Bosshart, J. T., & Bertolli, J. (2013). Shifting the paradigm: Using HIV surveillance data as a foundation for 225 improving HIV care and preventing HIV infection. *Milbank Quarterly, 91*(3), 558–603

Szent-Gyorgyi, L. E., Desai, S., Kim, D., Sax, P. E., & Greenberg, J. O. (2012). Removing legal barriers to high-quality care for HIV infected patients. *The New England Journal of Medicine, 366*, 1268–1270. https://www.nejm.org/doi/full/10.1056/NEJMp1114446

Tabachnick, B. G.& Fidell, L. S. (2013). *Using multivariate statistics* (6th ed). London: Pearson.

Teng, Y., & Mak, W. W. S. (2011). The role of planning and self-efficacy in condom use among men who have sex with men: An application of the health action process approach model. *Health Psychology 30*(1), 119–128.

Uccelli, M. M., Traversa, S., & Ponzio, M. (2016). A survey study comparing young adults with MS and healthy controls on self-esteem, self-efficacy, mood and quality of life. *Journal of the Neurological Sciences*, *368*, 369–373.

Ulrike, S., Walmsey, S., Monforte, A., & Johnson, M. (2013). Caring for women living with HIV: Gaps in the evidence. *Journal of the International AIDS Society, 16*(1), 331–338. https://doi.org/10.7448/IAS.16.1.18509 United States Census Bureau. (2017a). *Quick facts: Palm Beach Gardens city, Florida- population estimates*. https://www.census.gov

United States Census Bureau. (2017b). *Quick facts San Diego County, California* https://www.census.gov/quickfacts/fact/table/sandiegocountycalifornia,ca/PST045217

Warren-Findlow, J., Seymour, R. B., & Huber, L. R. B. (2012). The association between self-efficacy and hypertension self-care activities among African American adults. *Journal of Community Health*, *37*(1), 15–24.

Weinstein, N. D. (1988). The precaution adoption process. *Health Psychology*, 7(4), 355.

Wideman, L., Noar, S. M., Choukas-Bradley, S., & Francis, D. B. (2014). Adolescent sexual health communication and condom use: A meta-analysis. *Health Psychology*, 33(10), 1113.

World Health Organization. (2017). *Summary of the global HIV epidemic* http://www.who.int/hiv/data/2017_summaryglobal- hiv-epidemic.png?ua=1

Ybarra, M. L., Korchmaros, J., Kiwanuka, J., Bangsberg, D. R., & Bull, S. (2013). Examining the applicability of the IMB model in predicting condom use among sexually active secondary school students in Mbarara, Uganda. *AIDS and Behavior*, *17*(3), 1116–1128.

APPENDIX A: Letter Of Request

Dear ______________

I am writing to request your support for a research study addressing the health concerns of African American men. I am a doctoral student at Walden University, and this research is being conducted for a Ph.D. dissertation study entitled, "The Relationship between Self-Efficacy, Perceived Susceptibility and Condom Use Among African American Males". This study focuses on condom use as a sexually transmitted infection prevention method. The aim of this research is to provide insight to the health behaviors of African American men and ultimately impact disease prevention.

The research is anonymous; no identifying information will be requested. The research will consist of answering questionnaires and should require no more than 15 minutes of your time. We are specifically interviewing African American

Males ages 18- 35 who reside in the San Diego area of California. The research questions are of a sexual nature and resources will be provided for participants who may wish to seek additional information regarding sexual health. Please consider sharing the below Survey Monkey link with your membership so that they might allow their responses to aid this important research study.

Best Regards,
Karla Nash Ph.D.
Student,Walden University

APPENDIX B: Demographics Questionnaire

1. Age:
2. Highest Level of Education Completed
    a. Less than a High School Degree
    b. High School Graduate or GED
    c. Associates Degree
    d. Bachelor's Degree
    e. Advanced Degree

3. What is your sexual orientation?
    a. 2. Heterosexual
    b. 3. Gay
    c. 4. Bisexual
    d. 5. Other
4. What is the number of partners you have currently?

5. What is your frequency of sexual activity with others per week?
    a. 2. Less than once a week
    b. 3. One to three times a week
    c. 4. Four or more times a week

APPENDIX C: CUSES

CONDOM USE SELF-EFFICACY SCALE

The Condom Use Self-Efficacy Scale (CUSES) is a 28-item self-reported measure of one's personal ability to use condoms. Different aspects of condom use self-efficacy captured by the scale include individuals' feelings of confidence in the ability to access condoms, put on or take off a condom, and negotiate condom use. The estimated time for administration is 20 to 30 minutes.

ITEMS:

These questions ask about your own feelings about using condoms in specific situations. Please respond even if you are not sexually active or have never used (or had a partner who used) condoms. In such cases, indicate how you think you would feel in such a situation.

1. I feel confident in my ability to put a condom on myself or my partner.
2. I feel confident I could purchase condoms without feeling embarrassed.

3. I feel confident I could remember to carry a condom with me should I need one.
4. I feel confident in my ability to discuss condom usage with any partner I might have.
5. I feel confident in my ability to suggest using condoms with a new partner.
6. I feel confident I could suggest using a condom without my partner feeling "diseased."
7. I feel confident in my own or my partner's ability to maintain an erection while using a condom.
8. I would feel embarrassed to put a condom on myself or my partner.*
9. If I were to suggest using a condom to a partner, I would feel afraid that he or she would reject me.*
10. If I were unsure of my partner's feelings about using condoms, I would not suggest using one.*
11. I feel confident in my ability to use a condom correctly.
12. I would feel comfortable discussing condom use with a potential sexual partner before we ever had any sexual contact leg, hugging, kissing, caressing, etc.).
13. I feel confident in my ability to persuade a partner to accept using a condom when we have intercourse.

14. I feel confident I could gracefully remove and dispose of a condom after sexual intercourse.
15. If my partner and I were to try to use a condom and did not succeed, I would feel embarrassed to try to use one again (e.g., not being able to unroll condom, putting it on backwards, or awkwardness).*
16. I would not feel confident suggesting using condoms with a new partner because I would be afraid he or she would think I've had a past homosexual experience.*
17. I would not feel confident suggesting using condoms with a new partner because I would be afraid he or she would think I have a sexually transmitted disease.*
18. I would not feel confident suggesting using condoms with a new partner because I would be afraid he or she would think I thought they had a sexually transmitted disease.*
19. I would feel comfortable discussing condom use with a potential sexual partner before we ever engaged in intercourse.
20. I feel confident in my ability to incorporate putting a condom on myself or my partner into foreplay.
21. I feel confident that I could use a condom with a partner without "breaking the mood."
22. I feel confident in my ability to put a condom on myself or my partner quickly.

23. I feel confident I could use a condom during intercourse without reducing any sexual sensations.
24. I feel confident that I would remember to use a condom even after I have been drinking.
25. I feel confident that I would remember to use a condom even if I were high.
26. If my partner didn't want to use a condom during intercourse, I could easily convince him or her that it was necessary to do so.
27. I feel confident that I could use a condom successfully.
28. I feel confident I could stop to put a condom on myself or my partner even in the heat of passion.

*Items reverse coded during scoring Response Options:

Strongly agree = 0

Disagree = 1 Undecided = 2 Agree = 3 Strongly agree = 4

APPENDIX D: Perceived Risk Scale

STD Risk Assessment Questionnaire: Questions are multiple choice questions which will be coded numerically for analysis (see the parenthetical code following the response).

Scores range from 3 to 45.

Combine with Section E for a score range from 3 to 53.

1. Have you been seen in an STD clinic before?

a. (select one)

b. Yes (1)

c. No (0)

2. What was the reason for visiting an STD clinic?

(check all that apply)

a. Have symptoms (5)

b. Think you could be at risk for an STD/HIV (5)

c. No symptoms –STD testing/screening only (1)

d. Someone told you to come today (2)

e. Referred by another doctor or clinic (3)

a. Other (0)

3. Have you had sexual intercourse (vaginal, oral, or anal intercourse) in the last 6 months? (select one)

a. Yes (1)

b. No (0)

4. When with new or non-steady partners, do you use a condom or barrier? (select one)

a. Always (1)

b. Most of the time (2)

c. Sometimes (3)

d. Rarely (4)

e. Never (5)

5 Have you ever exchanged drugs/money for sex?

a. Yes (1)

b. No (0)

*Research has indicated that these behaviors demonstrate potentially high STD risk.

6. Have you ever engaged in sexual intercourse with a partner with a recent history of incarceration?

a. Yes (1)

b. No (0)

* Research has indicated that these behaviors demonstrate potentially high STD risk.

7. Do you smoke cigarettes?

a. Yes (1)

b. No (0)

* Research has indicated that these behaviors demonstrate potentially high STD risk.

8. Have you had sex with: (select one)

a. Man

b. Woman

c. Both Other

9. Have you had sex with someone you know injects

recreational drugs? (select one)

a. Yes

b. No

10. Have you had sex with someone you know has any other STD? If yes, which STD (select all that apply)

a. Chlamydia

b. Herpes

c. Trichomonas

d. Gonorrhea

e. NGU/NSU

f. HIV

g. Genital Warts

h. Syphilis

i. Not listed. Please fill in: ____________________

j. Do not know

11. Have you ever been diagnosed with an STD? (mark all that apply)

a. Chlamydia

b. Herpes

c. Trichomonas

d. Gonorrhea

e. NGU/NSU

f. HIV

g. Genital Warts

h. Syphilis

i. Not listed. Please fill in: ________________

j. Do not know

12. Have you ever been diagnosed with an STD more than 1 time? If yes, check all that apply below (mark all that apply)

a. Chlamydia

b. Herpes

c. Trichomonas

d. Gonorrhea

e. NGU/NSU

f. HIV

g. Genital Warts

h. Syphilis

i. Not listed. Please fill in: ____________________

j. Do not know

13. What is your primary reason for using condoms?

(select one)

a. STD Prevention

b. Pregnancy Prevention

c. I don't use condoms

APPENDIX E: Locations of Flyer Distribution in San Diego, CA

1. Gentry's Barber Shop –San Diego, CA 92113

2. Butta Cutz-San Diego, CA 92102

3. Legendz Barbershop -La Mesa, CA 91942

4. Jackie Robinson YMCA - San Diego, CA 92102

5. Mountain View Rec Center -San Diego, CA 92113

6. Skyline Hills Rec Center - San Diego, CA 92114

7. Bayview Baptist Church - San Diego, CA 92114

8. New Creation Church -San Diego, CA 92105

9. City of Hope Church -San Diego, CA 92113

10. Greater Apostolic Faith Temple- San Diego, CA 92102

APPENDIX F: Flyer With Tear-off Information

African American Males Research Study

Share your experience

We are inviting African American Men age 18-35 to participate in a research questionnaire.
Your participation will contribute to a research study on African American Men and their experience with HIV AIDS prevention methods.

Complete a 5.10-minute survey online from the comfort of your own home.
Your participation is anonymous and your responses will only be presented as an aggregate.
This research study is designed to advance knowledge of disease prevention.

For more info contact

Confidential Survey PHD Research Project Focus on disease prevention

African American Males
AfricanAmericanResearch@gmail.com
619-777-7777
www.research.com

African American Males
AfricanAmericanResearch@gmail.com
619-777-7777
www.research.com

African American Males
AfricanAmericanResearch@gmail.com
619-777-7777
www.research.com

African American Males
AfricanAmericanResearch@gmail.com
619-777-7777
www.research.com

African American Males
AfricanAmericanResearch@gmail.com
619-777-7777
www.research.com

African American Males
AfricanAmericanResearch@gmail.com
619-777-7777
www.research.com

APPENDIX G: Online Flyer Distribution

Digital posting on Facebook, Instagram, Twitter and other Social Media websites will be posted online:

Researcher seeks African American Males ages 18-35 who reside in California for a research study. The research questionnaire focuses on condom use as a sexually transmitted infection prevention method and will take no more than 15 minutes. The aim of this research is to provide insight to the health behaviors of African American men and ultimately impact disease prevention.

Please consider sharing the below Survey Monkey link to aid this important research study.

www.surveymonkey.com/StudyLink

APPENDIX H: Permission To Use CUSES Instrument

Request to Utilize CUSES Instrument in Research Study

You replied on Thu 12/3/2020 10:58 PM Wed 12/2/2020 9:01 AM

To: Karla Nash

The Condom Self-Efficacy Scale.docx

14 KB

Dear Ms. Nash,

You have my permission to use the CUSES in your dissertation research. It sounds very interesting.

I have attached a copy of it, along with scoring instructions. I would be interested in your results when they are ready to be released. Best wishes.

Kenneth H. Beck, Ph.D., FAAHB Professor Emeritus Department of Behavioral & Community Health School of Public Health University of Maryland College Park 20742.

APPENDIX I: Permission for Use of Perceived Risk Scale

Request for Use of Perceived Risk of HIV Scale

Fri 12/4/2020 9:16 AM

To: Karla Nash

Hi Karla,

Sorry for my slow response. We are in the middle of wrapping up classes for the semester. You have my permission to use the scale and include it in your thesis.

Good luck with your project!

Dr. Lucy Napper Associate Professor
Psychology Department
Health, Medicine, and Society Program
Chandler-Ullmann 107
Lehigh University

Self-Efficacy and Perceived Susceptibility as Predictors of Condom Use Among African American Males